The Practitioner/Teacher Role:
Practice What You Teach

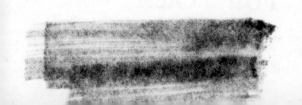

THE PRACTITIONER/ TEACHER ROLE:
Practice What You Teach

Edited by
LORRAINE MACHAN, R.N., Ph.D.
Professor
College of Nursing
Marquette University
Milwaukee, Wisconsin

This volume was selected for inclusion in the
NURSING DIMENSIONS EDUCATION SERIES
Volume I, Number 3, 1980

8 3 0 8

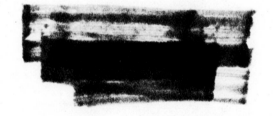

Table of Contents

List of Contributors

MARGARET BASTEYNS, Assistant Professor, College of Nursing, Marquette University, Milwaukee, Wisconsin

MARY E. CONWAY, Dean and Professor, School of Nursing, University of Wisconsin, Milwaukee, Wisconsin

LUTHER CHRISTMAN, Vice President Nursing Affairs and Dean, College of Nursing, Rush University, Chicago, Illinois

JEAN WOUTERS DiMOTTO, Assistant Professor, College of Nursing, Marquette University, Milwaukee, Wisconsin

LAURIE K. GLASS, Assistant Professor, School of Nursing, University of Wisconsin, Milwaukee, Wisconsin

PENNY J. GOODYEAR, Practitioner-Teacher, Marquette University, Milwaukee, Wisconsin

HELEN HARRINGTON, Associate Professor, College of Nursing, Marquette University, Milwaukee, Wisconsin

LORETTA KLASSEN, Assistant Professor, College of Nursing, Marquette University, Milwaukee, Wisconsin

LORRAINE MACHAN, Professor, College of Nursing, Marquette University, Milwaukee, Wisconsin

JUDITH FITZGERALD MILLER, Assistant Professor, College of Nursing, Marquette University, Milwaukee, Wisconsin

BETTY A. ROBERTS, Assistant Professor, School of Nursing, Fort Hays State University, Hays, Kansas

JOANNE S. STEVENSON, Associate Professor, Assistant Director for Research, and Director, Center for Nursing Research, Ohio State University, Columbus, Ohio

MADELINE MUSANTE WAKE, Director of Continuing Education and Assistant Professor, College of Nursing, Marquette University, Milwaukee, Wisconsin

A. LORRAINE WALLENBORN, Associate Professor, College of Nursing, Marquette University, Milwaukee, Wisconsin

Acknowledgments

The editor gratefully acknowledges the publisher of *The Journal of Nursing Administration* for permission to reprint the articles by Joanne S. Stevenson, which appear as Chapters 7 and 8 in Part II, and the publishers of *Nursing Outlook* for permission to reprint as Chapter 6 in Part II the article by Mary E. Conway and Laurie K. Glass.

Many of the ideas and developments described in this book were made possible by a three-year grant from the Division of Nursing, Department of Health, Education and Welfare for the project, 5 D23 NU 00038, Expanding a Role-Oriented Model for Graduate Education (1976-1979).

The editor also acknowledges Dean Rosalie Klein, Marquette University College of Nursing, for reviewing the chapters pertaining to curriculum to validate accuracy of content.

We wish it were possible to acknowledge by name the students whose contributions appear in Chapter 10 by Klassen and DiMotto. They know, nevertheless, that their permisson to use excerpts of their work is deeply appreciated.

A very special expression of thanks to Debra J. Bergeson, who typed several drafts of this manuscript into its final form and served as the secretary of the three-year project that led to this book.

Lorraine Machan
Milwaukee, Wisconsin
July 1979

All author royalties from sale of this book are consigned to a Marquette University Practitioner/Teacher Research Fund.

Preface

The stated purposes of this book are (1) to provide nurse educators with a concept of the Practitioner/Teacher as a multifaceted role that has the potential for improving patient care as well as nursing education and leads to fuller satisfaction in the professional role; (2) to describe the function of interagency collaboration in the successful implementation of the practitioner/teacher position; (3) to discuss role implementation problems and how some of them have been resolved; and (4) to describe the educational preparation of the practitioner/teacher through a role-oriented graduate program.

At this point in time when health care and education costs are soaring, the role of nurse educator obviously needs to be examined. The nursing profession as a whole has become acutely aware of the problems resulting from the separation of service and education. And, in efforts to attain the status of academicians for nurse-educators, the significance of this role as a practice discipline as well has not been given the attention it deserves. At the same time, many practicing nurses and administrators have failed to recognize the importance of developing nursing on a scientific base. It is also true that it is not unusual to find, in many hospitals, nurses with the title Clinical Specialist, who carry no caseload of patients—right here in the service setting the master practitioner is stripped of a practice role.

While the movement toward doctoral degree programs in nursing is gaining momentum, one can ask whether graduates of these programs are reducing or widening the gap between practice and education. This gap will not be closed until it can be demonstrated that practice, with research inherent in it, is a vital component of the teaching role.

This book has been developed largely from the efforts of a small group of faculty who served as team members for the federally funded project *Expanding a Role-Oriented Model for Graduate Education* (H.E.W. Grant No. 5 D23 NU00038-03). With a strong commitment to preparing advanced nursing practitioners at the Master's level and a long history of interest in educating quality teachers of nursing, it is not surprising that a program devoted to the development of the practitioner/teacher should emerge at this university.

It is our hope that this book will be instrumental in helping some of the many nurse educators now without a practice and/or research role, to find ways of implementing practice, with research as part of that practice, into their faculty function. We also hope it will inspire some clinical specialists to find ways of developing a full professional role as practitioner/teachers in service settings.

The educational model presented can be modified for program development at any level, including in-service and academic settings.

I
Practitioner/Teacher Models

Introduction

Lorraine Machan

The relatively rapid changes in professional nursing have brought with them, not surprisingly, problems for nurse educators. Within the past two decades a movement to unite or, as some might prefer, reunite practice and education has been perceptible. The successful unification efforts, through joint or shared appointments at the University of Florida, Case Western Reserve, and the University of Rochester, have been described by Powers (1976).[1] Many of us, however, have colleagues who entered joint appointments with enthusiasm and a year or two later found themselves exhausted from what they describe as two full-time jobs for the salary of one and the distinct impression that they were serving two masters, both of whom believed the other was getting the better end of the deal.

The presentations in Part One focus on models that appear to solve some of the problems of trying to bring practice and education together.

It is appropriate that the first chapter of this book is Luther Christman's working paper for Rush faculty. The Rush model provides a setting that frees the practitioner/teacher from the problems of serving two masters. Early in the development of our graduate program as a role-oriented model, a discussion with a Rush practitioner/teacher led me to believe that the goals of our program would prepare our graduate students to function in a role setting like that at Rush, which recognized how important it is for educators to maintain a practice role. A two-day visit to Rush by four of our graduate program faculty left all of us with the impression that something great was happening; that in spite of problems, which were discussed openly, the overwhelming response of the many people we spoke with was that each year had brought so much improvement over the previous ones they had to be optimistic and enthusiastic. Inspired by what

3

we had seen, but aware that we could not expect our university to buy a hospital, we looked for other types of settings in which practitioner/ teachers could function, not as joint or dual appointments but as one multi-faceted role.

It was, in fact, Christman who convinced me, perhaps unknown to himself, that only when the practitioner/teacher's role was viewed as a complex one rather than as two separate roles, would some of the problems associated with uniting teaching and practice be resolved.

The importance of administrative support from both education and service for the role to succeed is brought out in the remaining chapters of Part I. These chapters represent practitioner/teachers in three different settings and at three different levels of role development. Solutions to implementation problems, or methods used to prevent problems, are described, and the benefits resulting for patients, students, and the practitioner/teachers themselves are identified.

The reader will be able to see in the three examples, the progression in the perception of and movement toward a full faculty role.[2]

REFERENCES

1. Powers, Marjorie J.: The unification model in nursing. *Nursing Outlook,* 24:482–487, August 1976.
2. Barley, Zoe A. and Redman, Barbara K.: Faculty role development in university Schools of Nursing. *Journal of Nursing Administration,* 9:43–47, May 1979.

1
The Practitioner/Teacher
A Working Paper for the Faculty at Rush University College of Nursing and Allied Health Sciences*

Luther Christman

The practitioner/teacher role is an organizational device that is constructed to enable a professional practitioner to play the full professional role. The full professional role encompasses the subrole segments of service, education, consultation, and research. It is the expectation of society that professional persons will use this full role, in all its variations, in return for the society that accords the rights and privileges of professional status. Furthermore, students are helped, to a very great extent, by having viable behavioral models, when the full role is played, that smooths the way for a much more precise role socialization into the profession.

The basic conceptual design is illustrated in Figure 1.1.

The full expression of the practitioner/teacher role is contingent upon an organizational format that best facilitates the utilization of the full content of the role. The organizational structure should reduce role ambiguity to a minimum. The structure also should be a safeguard against role deprivation. Role deprivation (Bennis et al, 1961) can be defined as either violation

---

*This paper was originally written to assist the faculty to understand the practitioner-teacher role because of the general lack of that model in the nursing profession. The author has often acknowledged the utilization of this type of role in the education of clinical psychologists, veterinarians, dentists, physicians, and podiatrists where it has demonstrated its strength and productivity.

As described, the practitioner-teacher is a broad and adaptable role. It varies in degree of direct and indirect application. At the direct care level, where practitioner-teachers share their patients with their students, it is most visible. At levels where administrative components are necessary, it is less direct and visible. However, the level of the faculty clinical investigative studies, clinical electives, and directed study all have simlar visibility and expose a wide range of behavior models.

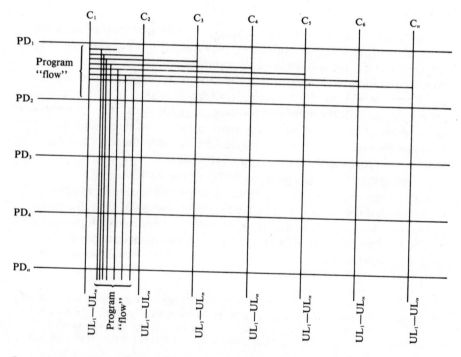

C = chairperson, PD = program director, UL = unit leader.

Fig. 1.1 Matrix-model organization of human resources and their interactions.

of anticipated role expression or failure to meet the expectations of the persons enacting the role. The use of a matrix type organization design is an effective means of achieving these objectives. The organization of the College of Nursing and Allied Health Sciences is in this pattern.

The chairpersons have line authority and are responsible and accountable for managing the resources allocated in order to achieve the goals and aspirations of their respective departments. Chairpersons must monitor all the professional efforts of their departments to ascertain that the professional standards of that specialty are being met and that the standards conform to the expectations of the University. Chairpersons, in addition, must give watchful attention to the interdigitation of their department with other departments of the College, to departments in other Colleges of the University, and to management in general.

Program directors have line authority and are responsible and accountable for managing the successful conduct of the specific programs to which they are assigned. Programs may be internal to a department or cut across two or more departments. Program directors, moreover, must give special attention to the interface of their programs with all other College and/or University programs to insure the best possible use of resources.

Unit leaders are the same prototype of management to their respective units as are chairpersons to their departments.

The crucial interactions in the matrix model occur at any point where a chairperson, unit leader, program director, and teacher/practitioners converge. The sum total of the nature of these interactions predict how successful the organization will be carrying out its goals.

The participants in a matrix type model may be viewed as professional free agents. To be effective, the free agent model must be seen as self-direction without anarchy. The matrix model provides a means of organizing human resources in such a way as to permit the optimum facilitation of each role. This concept implies that reasonable trade-offs take place to permit the system to be managed so that all participants, in all the various roles, experience a high degree of professional achievement and professional satisfaction.

A chairperson must manage the position responsibilities in a way that attracts and retains willing participants in the department. Chairpersons have to develop organizational climates within their departments that are conducive to this end. This same set of characteristics applies to the unit leader at the unit level.

Program directors must manage their position in a fashion that retains willing participants in each specific program. Faculty members must have a sense of professional excitement in participating in the program to maintain a keen interest in them and to generate the zest necessary to keep the programs productive.

Practitioner/teachers must be competent, both professionally and interpersonally, in order to be invited to join a department or a program. If practitioner/teachers do not demonstrate the required proficiency and other desirable role attributes, they will be unattractive to program directors, chairpersons, and unit leaders.

The foregoing brief statements illustrate the possibilities and limitations of the free-agent role. When the total system of a matrix type organization and free agent role are working in a harmonious balance, the possibility of attaining role certainty is at its best. The system, when finely tuned, is practically self-regulating.

Some assumptions always must be made when talking about role clarification in a health university. For example, one must assume that the curriculum for each college has faculty involvement and concurrence and that each educational program is on target. Another assumption worthy of primary consideration is that each practitioner/teacher is *teaching on his/her own set of patients*. Each practitioner/teacher is sharing the patients with the students while teaching. This is an essential condition because it is basic to the economy of effort required to play the full professional role. Violation of this principle will lead to a great deal of role strain. As each new assumption is stated its implication for organizational climate can be delineated.

This brief paper has been prepared as a working document to lay out a base for faculty deliberation regarding the role of the practitioner/teacher.

REFERENCE

Bennis, W.G., Berkowitz, N.H., Malone, M.F., and Klein, M.K.: *The Role of the Nurse in the Outpatient Department: A Preliminary Report.* The American Nurses' Foundation: New York, 1961.

2
Developing the Practitioner/Teacher Role in a Private Hospital Setting

Margaret Basteyns

In recent years, several clinical specialists have discussed in the literature their duties and responsibilities in joint appointments. Campbell (1970) was the first to relate how, as a "joint appointee," she "combined the responsibilities of faculty member at the University of Wisconsin School of Nursing and supervisor at the University Hospital."[1] Alexander (1972) described how she combined "full-time teaching and part-time practice" while employed as a faculty member of a pediatric-nurse/practitioner program.[2] In 1973, Vaughan analyzed her "triple appointment" as a nurse clinical specialist in pediatrics, a therapist in an outpatient department of child and adolescent psychiatry, and a member of a college of nursing graduate program in psychiatry.[3]

All of the authors concluded that functioning in a joint appointment was valuable. One summarized the value as threefold: "It is (1) beneficial to the students to have a person with a high degree of clinical competence as an instructor; (2) beneficial to the clinical specialist to keep up in the field; and (3) beneficial to both the hospital and the teaching institution by providing liaison relationships and continuity of knowledge and practice."[4]

Campbell and Vaughan presented their positions mainly from the viewpoint of clinical specialists. Because there is a growing concern among nursing school faculty over how to maintain their clinical expertise in fast-changing health care settings, this chapter examines the joint appointment once again, but with more emphasis on the faculty segment of such a position.

It should be clarified at the outset that the writer does not refer to her position of practitioner/teacher as a joint appointment. That term seems to connote functioning in two distinct roles or working in two part-time jobs, e.g., one in the hospital and another in a school of nursing. My practi-

9

tioner/teacher position involves only one role, which I consider multi-dimensional. The only manner in which a division exists in my position is that payment of my salary is divided between the school and the agency.

Some common threads are essential to weaving my practitioner/teacher role into one. Those threads are the patients, the nursing students, and the clinical setting. This means that the responsibility for the care of some patients to whom I give care as a practitioner is transferred to the students in the clinical area and vice versa. Secondly, my duties as a clinical instructor are fulfilled on the same hospital units in which I function as a practitioner so that the personnel with whom I work and the physical surroundings are constant elements.

IMPLEMENTATION OF THE ROLE OF PRACTITIONER/TEACHER

The nature of the position of practitioner/teacher defies writing a clear-cut job description. The role of the clinical specialist is continually evolving, and I find my role of practitioner/teacher equally evolutionary. The possibilities for creative teaching and improving patient care are overwhelming at times, and priorities are continually being reset. As one writer aptly stated: "Probably the most difficult and therefore confusing aspect of role development is establishing goals and objectives that are attainable."[5]

The simplest way for me to outline how a practitioner/teacher position can be developed and implemented is by describing my duties and responsibilities during a typical 10-month academic year.

The Dean of the College of Nursing, where I am employed as an Assistant Professor, initiated my contract with the Assistant Administrator in charge of Nursing Service at a 391-bed general hospital. This contract stated that the university would pay two-thirds of my salary and the hospital would contribute the other one-third. The basis of my practitioner/teacher position then was a mutual financial agreement between the university and the agency.

In return for the hospital's contribution to my salary, it was specified by the Assistant Administrator that I would be expected to spend an average of 13 hours a week in service as a practitioner. It was not stated in the contract how or on which unit in the hospital I was to function. These elements were negotiable, for which I was very grateful. As MacPhail (1971) pointed out when describing the mode of operation selected by the nurse clinician: "An essential condition is willingness of the employer to permit development of a role that differs from traditional roles in nursing. In addition, the nurse clinican needs freedom to define the role and formulate objectives and means of attaining them."[6]

My main responsibility at the College of Nursing is the clinical guidance and instruction of a group of six junior nursing students and four senior students at the same hospital where I would be working as a practitioner. All of these students are assigned to practice on the same 54-bed general medical unit. The juniors spend 12½ hours in the clinical area on Tuesdays and Wednesdays, while the seniors average 16 hours of practice each week, spread over Tuesday, Wednesday, and Thursday. Both the Fall and Spring semesters require 14 weeks of clinical practice. Each senior spends an average of 4 of those weeks off the assigned unit for experience in critical care and emergency room nursing.

Besides preparation for, participation in, and evaluation of the students' clinical practice, I have other responsibilities at the college. I am expected to attend both junior and senior level Care of the Adult faculty meetings once a month, be present at the general faculty meeting once a month, and participate in pertinent course-planning meetings held three to four times a year. I was also named chairperson of one of the college's standing committees, which requires monthly meetings.

After some discussion with the junior and senior level course coordinators and an assessment of my clinical instruction area and responsibilities, I decided where and how I would like to serve in the hospital. I wanted to carry out my practitioner role by working in a staff nurse position in the hospital's 12-bed mixed medical-surgical ICU. Several factors prompted this decision. First of all, the 14 senior nursing students assigned to this hospital are expected to get at least 16 hours of experience in this ICU without direct supervision or guidance from an instructor. Students had voiced dissatisfaction and boredom with this experience in previous years because it was mainly an observational one. The ICU staff, in turn, was uncomfortable and defensive because they knew the students were bored, but the nurses were hesitant to let them get too involved in patient care without an instructor in the immediate area. I thought that by working in ICU, I would get to know the staff and could then discern which of them felt the most comfortable with students. I would also be able to make better judgments about appropriate patients for whom senior students could provide care and could then structure their experience more closely.

Another reason for electing to work in the ICU was that 15-20 percent of these patients are eventually transferred to the medical unit where junior and senior students have their general clinical practice. My working in ICU would therefore make it possible to provide some continuity in the care of these patients after they left the unit, which can be helpful for any acutely ill person.

Finally, intensive care nursing had been my area of expertise during 6 of my 8 years of staff nursing. I hoped to continue using the skills I had acquired and to increase my knowledge in this field of nursing.

The Assistant Administrator in charge of Nursing Service was very open to my ideas and most agreeable as to my method of operation as well as the unit on which I wished to practice.

Strategies Used to Implement the Practitioner/Teacher Role

Since I had not worked at this hospital or with any of its personnel previously, I thought the best way to become familiar with the system was to go through the four-week orientation program held for all newly hired nurses. In the course of this orientation period I worked ten eight-hour shifts in ICU and five eight-hour shifts on the general medical unit where the students would be assigned. Through this program, I met key personnel in the hospital, became aware of the most important nursing service and major department policies and procedures, and became acquainted with most of the nursing personnel with whom I would be working on a day-to-day basis. All of this knowledge was not only helpful, but I felt it was essential information that would enable me to establish a base from which I could function as a practitioner/teacher in that hospital.

I found the ICU and medical unit head nurses and staff nurses very open and they accepted me as a person and a practitioner. These nurses, particularly those in ICU, were somewhat confused, however, about how I would be carrying out this practitioner/teacher position when school started. Most of the ICU nurses viewed me simply as holding two jobs. So during coffee and lunch breaks, I discussed informally the contract that had been drawn up between the university and the hospital, what my specific responsibilities were, and also outlined some of my objectives. The importance of making known to all who work consistently with the person that the practitioner/teacher's role is a dual position cannot be overemphasized. If the practitioner/teacher does not communicate the duties and objectives of the role, misunderstandings, confusion, and serious morale problems could result.

There were no problems in establishing rapport with the personnel on either of these units. The staff on the medical unit is accustomed to students and clinical instructors and at first communicated with me as though teaching was my only role. Shortly after I completed the orientation program, however, a number of the nurses observed me functioning also as a practitioner. Some received reports from me on patients being transferred from ICU, or vice versa. Others worked side by side with me when I was assigned to their unit during slow periods in ICU. These incidents caused them to consult and discuss with me, as a colleague, various patient care problems and strategies. Many eventually did this on a regular basis, and yet they were always respectful of the fact that when the students were present, my time and primary responsibility was for the students.

I anticipated having some difficulty in getting established and becoming an insider in ICU. I therefore scheduled myself to work at least one Saturday and occasionally one complete weekend a month. This was my way of nonverbally letting the staff know that I was aware of their working situation and that I did not feel I was above all that. This strategy worked well and after I proved myself to be a hard worker and a good nurse, the ICU nurses also started to use me as a consultant and resource person. While I continued doing the work of a staff nurse when on duty in the ICU, I was in time considered to be more than that. My responsibilities were not expanded, but how I functioned and how I was utilized definitely did expand.

Problems in Implementing the Practitioner/Teacher Role

What has been stated above may make it seem as though things couldn't have gone more smoothly, but some problems did arise. During the first few months, there was a good deal of frustration at times.

One problem I had to deal with in the beginning was getting phone calls at home from various nursing service supervisors at the hospital. They either wanted to know if I could work the evening or night shift in ICU for someone who could not come in or they needed extra help on the weekend. This was a clue to me that while my position was known to the key people in the Nursing Office and to the ICU Head Nurse, it was not clear to the supervisors who took over when they were not there. To these people, I was just another part-time nurse on the employee roster, and they saw no reason not to call me. After the third phone call in one week, I discussed this matter with the supervisor in charge of ICU. She understood my situation very well and after she made a special notation on my card in the nursing office, I received no further phone calls or requests to work hours or days for which I was not scheduled.

Another problem that arose in the course of the Fall semester was that the junior students felt I was not giving them enough of my time. This feeling was precipitated mainly by the fact that I left the medical unit 45 minutes to an hour on Tuesdays and Wednesdays to check on the seniors who were doing clinical practice in ICU. Even though I did not leave the juniors until late in the morning when they were involved with their patient care, they still felt slightly neglected and insecure without me there. The solution to this dilemma was suggested by some of the nurses in ICU. If the seniors could be scheduled for clinical practice on Thursdays, why not place them in ICU on that day instead of Tuesday or Wednesday? Since I worked almost every Thursday in ICU, the students would be able to work with me and I would not have to neglect the juniors in any way. I presented this suggestion to the Nursing Service Director, the Supervisor of ICU, and the Head Nurse. They felt that having the senior students in the unit on Thursdays would create no problem. This plan was initiated in the Spring semester. It proved to be an ideal solution to the time-conflict with the juniors. For the seniors the ICU experience became one of the highlights of their semester.

A source of frustration, especially during the early months of my working in this practitioner/teacher position, was not being able to make full use of my knowledge or talents when working in the ICU. I am capable of functioning as a clinical specialist but had chosen not to do so for several reasons. First of all, there are two clinical specialists already associated with the ICU. They involve themselves with the intensive care patients, either after making their own assessment of them or after being called for consultation by one of the staff. That 12-bed unit did not need another person functioning mainly as a clinical specialist.

Another reason for not working in that role was that patient care involvement during my 13 hours of service would have been very sporadic. If there were no consultations or patient care difficulties during the shift I scheduled myself to practice, what would I do with my time? I could quickly be viewed as an intruder if I asked to take care of some patients just to keep myself occupied.

A second factor contributing to my frustrations was that I felt it necessary to be "low key" while working in ICU until I had established myself. I was not only a new staff person, but was in a new and different position and the personnel had a need and a right to "feel me out." If I had been too aggressive in my interpersonal relations or constantly offering unsolicited advice, ideas, or opinions about patient care or staff problems, I would have alienated the other nurses. Gradually, as the nurses learned to know me and heard my discussions with students, they too began to use me as a resource person and as a teacher. I am no longer "just another worker." But, this took time, and during that time I had to deal with the knowledge that I was capable of doing and being more.

Potential Difficulties in Implementing a Practitioner/Teacher Role

Before leaving the subject of implementation of the role of practitioner/ teacher, some possible pitfalls and deterring factors to such implementation should be mentioned. The need for good communication between one's superiors, as well as their support and understanding, should be reemphasized. This point has been made numerous times in the literature with regard to the clinical specialist.[7] This position should be initiated and established by the appropriate administrators at the school and the agency. The obligations and expectations placed on the person chosen for a practitioner/teacher position need to be outlined and understood also. Guidelines should not be set so rigidly that they eliminate creativity and flexibility; however, the broad objectives of what each institution wants to accomplish through the person they have jointly employed need to be clearly understood by all involved.

A major complication in fulfilling a combined position could occur if one aspect of the role places too much responsibility on the person. For example, one might be asked to function as a Head Nurse or Assistant Head Nurse at the hospital, or as a Course Coordinator at the school. Trying to combine the work of a clinical instructor with that of Assistant Head Nurse could be confusing to the personnel with whom one is working on a daily basis. The bigger problem, however, would be exhaustion and frustration over trying to accomplish too much in the course of one week. The duties and responsibilities of a part-time Assistant Head Nurse or of a Course Coordinator cannot generally be carried out in a fixed amount of time every pay period. Such a position requires some flexibility in hours so that more or less time can be given as necessary to various responsibilities. In order to compensate and attempt to find more time when it is needed, a person in such a role will use hours they should either be giving to another part of their position or they dip into time that should be used for personal obligations, learning, and recreation. Thus, if one segment of a multidimensional appointment requires playing a very responsibility-laden role, the person will gradually burn out physically, and lose objectivity and enthusiasm.

THE BENEFITS OF WORKING IN A COMBINED PRACTITIONER/TEACHER ROLE

After working in a practitioner/teacher position for 10 months, I was aware that the advantages of such an appointment greatly outnumbered any disadvantages. There were definite benefits that had accrued to the nursing students, to the patients, to the nursing staff, and to myself as the practitioner/teacher that were a direct result of my functioning in this multidimensional role. Christman (1976) summarized those benefits by stating that:

> Practitioner-teachers are in an advantageous position to serve as link pins between the theory and content of science and its application to practice. By cooperating with students in clinical settings, they are behavioral models of expertise. . . . By acting as consultants to other nurses on the staff, practitioner-teachers can raise the quality of the overall endeavor.[8]

Benefits for the Students

Evaluations by both the junior and senior students consistently revealed that they felt the environment for learning in the clinical area was "excellent" and "growth producing." Being familiar with the hospital, key personnel in various departments, and major policies and procedures certainly affected my ability to create and maintain an atmosphere that was conducive to the students' learning. Likewise, the fact that I not only knew the nursing personnel on the medical unit and in ICU, but also worked with them, helped create better relations and promoted the sharing of ideas and more interaction between students and staff. The students stated that they felt "involved" and "a part of things" when they worked; they were not the "outsiders" they had been in some previous clinical facilities.

Another benefit for the students was pointed out by the seniors in relation to their ICU experience. They stated that their patient assignments while in that unit "correlated very well with their classroom theory." This circumstance was again a direct result of my working in ICU and thus knowing the patients and their problems.

Finally, all of the students remarked in varying ways and contexts that my evaluation of them and my views of nursing practice in the hospital setting were significant to them because they knew I was a practitioner as well as an instructor. They saw me as a role model of a practitioner. Several seniors mentioned that they valued what I said because they felt that I "really knew what it was going to be like in the world of work after they graduated."

Benefits for the Patients

The main benefit that accrued to a significant number of patients because of my combined position was continuity of their care. Most weeks, at least one patient assigned to a student had been transferred to the medical unit from ICU. Working in the ICU gave me direct knowledge of the patient and his problems, which I shared with the nursing staff and students.

At times the situation was reversed and patients on the medical unit required intensive care. Again I was able to share what I knew about the patient with the ICU staff and often gave personal care to these patients.

Continuity of patient care was also achieved to a more limited degree by some senior nursing students assigned for clinical practice with a different instructor on a 56-bed surgical unit. I guided and worked with these students during their ICU experience. They often worked with the same patients they had cared for in ICU when these patients were later transferred to the surgical unit.

With regard to the status of overall patient care, the Head Nurses of the Medical Unit and of the ICU both stated that they thought my activities had helped improve the quality of care being given on their units. I supported them in their management decisions and helped them work through some of the problems of initiating a Primary Nursing Care system. These Head Nurses also felt that through incidental discussions as well as more structured teaching sessions, I had assisted their staffs to improve their nursing knowledge and skills, and hopefully the patients benefited by this.

Benefits for the Nursing Staff

The staff in both ICU and the medical unit frequently used me as a resource person. They would consult with me mainly about patient care problems but at times they asked for my perspective on staff or administrative issues or problems as well. The awareness of my nursing experience by the various staff members and physicians of these units stemmed directly from my activities as a practitioner/teacher. They saw me in action not only teaching, but also giving direct patient care. This had a definite bearing on the degree to which personnel came to me to collaborate or ask for help. Some mentioned that because they knew I was a practitioner, they "were not afraid to approach me" to discuss problems or share ideas. The less experienced nurses, especially, felt I helped them through conversations, discussions, and demonstrations to integrate their knowledge, increase their confidence, and develop their nursing skills and strategies.

Personal Benefits for the Practitioner/Teacher

Working in a combined position gave me an opportunity to make the most of the assets and strengths I had developed in the area of nursing practice over a period of 10 years. I enjoy giving direct patient care and having some influence on the type of care being given. I also like being involved in the clinical instruction of others, whether it be staff or students. Being in a practitioner/teacher position allowed me to do both of these things. This is in contrast to a full-time faculty or hospital education position where the main responsibility is instruction of others. Hospital clinical specialists also do not usually have the opportunity to give direct patient care to the extent that I did.

Functioning in a practitioner/teacher role was an ideal way for me to maintain clinical competence while teaching nursing students. Methods of remaining current and abreast of the latest techniques in clinical nursing are often discussed among nursing school faculty. To work in a combined position is not the only solution to this common problem, but I found it a very rewarding and realistic one. Also, what better way is there to be a behavioral model to nursing students, not only of clinical expertise, but also of such attributes as curiosity, open-mindedness, flexibility, the capacity to think critically, and the need to take responsibility for one's continued learning?

SUMMARY

The writer has given an account of the dynamic process involved in establishing and carrying out her role of practitioner/teacher. Difficulties encountered and potential problems are described. There are many benefits attached to this position and they accrue to the nursing students, the patients, the nursing staff, and to the practitioner/teacher herself.

Establishing role identity and functioning as practitioner/teacher requires the same qualifications and characteristics expected of a clinical specialist. A sound nursing background obtained through several years of professional experience followed by a master's degree in nursing is essential. Desirable personal qualities are patience, tact, open-mindedness, objectivity, and flexibility. A spirit of adventure and creativity are also important because the role of both the clinician and the practitioner/teacher are evolutionary. These roles, as any role, are not set; instead, the person playing the part continually constructs and reconstructs the role in response to many factors.

An effort has been made in this discussion to focus on the practitioner/teacher position as one multidimensional role. Administrators of schools of nursing, in particular, must become aware of the need to create such a position among their faculty. It is one way for their members to maintain clinical expertise. More frequently, however:

If nurse educators decline to spend a large portion of their time in practice, standards of nursing care will be set by the next lower order of practicing nurses. Moreover, failure to practice means that educators are creating a major credibility gap for themselves, not only with nurses, but also with members of other professions (Christman 1976).[9]

REFERENCES

1. Campbell, Emily B.: The clinical nurse specialist: Joint appointee. *American Journal of Nursing,* 70:543–546, March 1970.
2. Alexander, Mary M.: Combining teaching with clinical practice. *Supervisor Nurse,* 3:13–17, June 1972.
3. Vaughan, Beth Ann: Role fusion, diffusion, and confusion. *Nursing Clinics of North America,* 8:703–713, December 1973.
4. Ibid.
5. Ibid.
6. MacPhail, Janetta: Reasonable expectations for the nurse clinician. *Journal of Nursing Administration,* 1:16–18, September–October 1971.
7. Shaefer, Jeanne A.: The satisfied clinician: Administrative support makes the difference. *Journal of Nursing Administration,* 3:17–20, July–August 1973; McFarland, Mary Brambilla: Adaptability in the nurse clinician role. *Supervisor Nurse,* 4:23–29, February 1973; MacPhail, Janetta: Reasonable expectations for the nurse clinician. *Journal of Nursing Administration,* 1:16–18, September–October 1971; Parkis, Ellen W: The management role of the clinical specialist, Part I. *Supervisor Nurse,* 5:44–51, September 1974; Parkis, Ellen W.: The management role of the clinical specialist, Part II. *Supervisor Nurse,* 5:24–35, October 1974.
8. Christman, Luther: Where are we going—an editorial. *Journal of Nursing Administration,* 6:15–16, February 1976.
9. Ibid.

Suggested Reading

Alexander, Mary M.: Combining teaching with clinical practice. *Supervisor Nurse,* 3: 13–17, June 1972.

Backsheider, Joan: The clinical nursing specialist as a practitioner. *Nursing Forum,* 10: 359–376, 1971.

Bivin, Victoria E.: The clinical specialist—an educator. *Nursing Clinics of North America,* 8: 715–722, December 1973.

Butts, Priscilla A.: The clinical specialist vs. the clinical supervisor. *Supervisor Nurse,* 5: 38–44, April 1974.

Campbell, Emily B.: The clinical nurse specialist: Joint appointee. *American Journal of Nursing,* 70:543–546, March 1970.

Christman, Luther: Where are we going—an editorial. *Journal of Nursing Administration,* 6:15–16, February 1976.

Conway, Mary E.: Management effectiveness and the role-making process. *Journal of Nursing Administration*, 4:25-28, November-December 1974.

Edwards, Jane: Clinical specialists are not effective—why? *Supervisor Nurse*, 2:39-47, August 1971.

MacPhail, Janetta: Reasonable expectations for the nurse clinician. *Journal of Nursing Administration*, 1:16-18, September-October 1971.

McFarland, Mary Brambilla: Adaptability in the nurse clinician role. *Supervisor Nurse*, 4: 23-29, February 1973.

McGann, Marlene Reuter: The clinical specialist: From hospital to clinic, to community. *Journal of Nursing Administration*, 5:33-36, March-April 1975.

Parkis, Ellen W.: The management role of the clinical specialist, Part I. *Supervisor Nurse*, 5: 44-51, September 1974.

Parkis, Ellen W.: The management role of the clinical specialist, Part II. *Supervisor Nurse*, 5: 24-35, October 1974.

Pearson, Linda E.: The clinical specialist as role model or motivator? *Nursing Forum*, (No. 1, 1972) 11:71-77.

Plawecki, Judith Ann: Viewpoint on the preparation of the clinical nurse specialist. *Supervisor Nurse*, 1:49-63, January 1971.

Shaefer, Jeanne A.: The satisfied clinician: Administrative support makes the difference. *Journal of Nursing Administration*, 3:17-20, July-August 1973.

Stevens, Barbara J.: Accountability of the clinical specialist: The administrator's viewpoint. *Journal of Nursing Administration*, 6:30-32, February 1976.

Vaughan, Beth Ann: Role fusion, diffusion, and confusion. *Nursing Clinics of North America*, 8:703-713, December 1973.

3
Health Clinics for the Elderly:
Practitioner/Teachers in a
Community Setting

Lorraine Machan and Betty Roberts

Nursing health clinics are being established in many areas throughout the United States. They range from fee-for-service to free; clinics conducted by independent nurse practitioners to clinics provided by various health agencies.[1] The clinic settings for the elderly that will be described in this chapter were established and are maintained by the community health faculty of Fort Hays State University School of Nursing, in Hays, Kansas. The faculty members who maintain the clinic exemplify the practitioner/ teacher role, incorporating practice, teaching, and research. The development of these clinics is an appropriate endorsement of Barley and Redman's (1979) view that "clinical practice is another area that can provide opportunities for faculty development, increased status, and inter-disciplinary relationships."[2]

The idea for the clinics grew from the strong community health emphasis in the baccalaureate program which developed as a model for a rural environment.[3]

The suggestion was made to Betty Roberts, who was pursuing a master's degree in nursing, that a suitable research project for her graduate program of study might be to carry out a feasibility study on the development of a faculty-maintained clinic for the elderly. On the basis of this study, the first clinic was established at a meal-site center for the elderly in November 1974. A second clinic was established in June 1977 at a high-rise apartment building for the elderly. Three faculty members share the responsibility for the full case load of clients. At the time of writing, this totals 240, of which 160 are meal-site clients and 80 are high-rise clients from 90 apartments. The clinic at each site is held one morning every two weeks, with sites alternating each week, but between clinics assistance is available for clients.

Phone calls from clients who need advice or have questions they want answered are quite frequent and even occasional home visits are made. Some of the clients have asked to have their names placed on the nursing school's home-visit schedule for students.

HOW THE CLINIC IS STAFFED AND OPERATED

Each clinic is staffed by two faculty members and five to six students. Thirty to 35 clients are cared for in a morning (four hours). Clients are seen by appointments which vary in frequency from every two weeks to once a month, or even once every six weeks. "Walk-ins" are also accepted, and the fact that no fuss is made if an appointment is not kept, has had favorable results. Records are kept on weight, blood pressure, pulse, respiration, sleep and exercise patterns, nutrition, and medications. Heart and lung assessments, breast exams, and hearing tests, along with other aspects of assessment, are carried out as needed. Assistance with understanding the medication regimen, and just listening to what clients have to say and providing appropriate emotional support are among the most important nursing functions carried out.

The nursing clinics have had the support and cooperation of the medical community. Clients are referred to their own physicians, as necessary, and physicians refer clients to the clinic. The clients are made very aware that the clinic is not a substitute for but an addition to the care provided by the physician. Each client has a small booklet of personal data in which both nurses and physicians write entries. Although there is no charge for the services, the clients understand that they are contributing by providing an educational experience for nursing students.

Equipment and supplies for the clinics are provided by the School of Nursing. The meal site and apartment management provide screens and lockable cabinets. Five examining booths are available during a clinic. The clinics are under the auspices of the School of Nursing of the University in conjunction with the meal-site center and Centennial Towers, the high-rise apartment. Both faculty and students carry liability insurance.

Additional time at the clinic sites on clinic days is used for lecture/demonstrations, discussion, and conference. For example, problem-oriented recording is taught as part of this experience, as is the use of some equipment, such as the audiometer, otoscope, and titmus machine. Only senior students are assigned to the clinics, since the faculty believes the foundation of the first three years is necessary. As much as possible, students follow the same clients. Each student participates in four to six clinics.

The case load of clients has not, to date, created problems with the teaching load, and the clinics have provided one very effective way for students to gain community health experience. This, of course, is not the only community health experience in the curriculum, but it is a setting that has provided faculty members with the opportunity for practice, teaching, and research.

Practitioner/Teacher Calvina Thomas conducted an attitude study in 1976 and recently did a follow-up study (1979). The study revealed that in both years attitudes of clients toward illness-prevention services were very positive. The clients also believe the nursing clinic has helped them, and about one-third of the clients reduced their needs to see a physician from once-a-month to once every three months. On clinic days, meal-site attendance increases by up to 20 persons.

Betty Roberts, collaborating with sociologist Rose Arnold, recently completed a project, "Congregate Housing for the Elderly: Reasons for and Expressed Satisfaction with Relocation." The interdisciplinary colleagueship that produced the research paper also resulted in a jointly taught course, the Sociology of Aging and Its Implications.

DO NURSING CLINICS PROVIDE BETTER CARE?

In addition to the results of Thomas's study, practitioner/teachers believe that their elderly clients have improved their health knowledge and feel more confident talking about medications and asking questions of physicians. They also appeared to be more self-assertive. Clients always carry their personal-data books with them, and one man was able to get help in an emergency situation because the nursing-clinic data book provided very useful information to help him through the crisis.

From the students' point of view, the clinic has provided them with more opportunity for independent action and nursing decisions. The school of nursing has approximately 40 graduates a year. In the four and one-half years since the first senior participants in 1974, only one student has indicated that she did not find the experience valuable. Students gained insight into primary care nursing and continuity of care. They also had the opportunity to organize and teach health programs, both to individuals and to groups. By federal directive, meal-site participants must receive at least six health programs a year. The students have been able to observe differences in the active elderly and those cared for in a nursing home, a setting for an earlier part of their program of study. Many students selected a clinic-related project for their research requirements, and two students, as a leadership project, assisted in the development of the clinic at the high-rise apartments.

The pride and enthusiasm these practitioner/teachers show with respect to their clinics leads one to believe them when they say that this setting for teaching, practice, and research has increased their satisfaction with their professional role. There has been an almost unbelievable scarcity of obstacles in the development and current maintenance of the clinics described above. Reflecting on the writings of nurse clinicians, one author states: "Generally all of these reports emphasize strong and open administrative support as a necessary component to the successful evolution of clinical roles."[4] There is no doubt that this type of administrative support has been one outstanding reason for the successful Fort Hays Clinics. These faculty members received support from the past and present nursing deans, university president, and county health officer, a medical doctor who took a recommendation supporting the development of the clinic to the County Medical Society. Another major reason for success has been the careful planning by a study (Roberts 1976) that assessed the health care needs of the population to be served by the clinics. Even after the pilot study was completed, faculty members initiating the project visited with the groups for at least two months before a clinic setting was established.

Sullivan (1978) writes about primary care providers,

. . . working collaboratively with other professionals and accepting a high degree of accountability for one's actions requires assertiveness and willingness to seek change in both one's self and the system of health care.[5]

Powers (1976) believes "new role incumbents . . . need a certain combination of fortitude, patience, prudence, and optimism in order to survive." I would add to this list of qualities, enthusiasm and a high level of commitment.

After the first Fort Hays clinic was established, the commitment to maintain continuity in meeting client needs between clinics has required sacrifices of some personal time from the practitioner/teachers who are willing to counsel by phone and make occasional home visits, as necessary. Calvina Thomas, with the assistance of students, volunteered her service for the entire first summer of clinic operation. These efforts have been rewarded by the satisfaction of a nurse/client relationship that has been mutually beneficial. The elderly citizens who are receiving better health care are very much aware of and take pride in the contribution they are making to the education of nursing students.

REFERENCES

1. Roberts, Betty: Feasibility of a nursing health clinic at the meal-site center in Hays, Kansas, a professional paper, Texas Woman's University, Graduate School, Dallas, Texas, 1976.
2. Barley, Zoe and Redman, Barbara: Faculty role development in university schools of nursing. *Journal of Nursing Administration,* 9:43–47, May 1979.
3. Machan, Lorraine: H.E.W. Planning Grant ID 10 NU09904-01 to Upgrade and Expand an Existing Baccalaureate Program to Meet National Accreditation Standards, Increase Student Enrollment, and Develop as a Model for a Rural Environment, 1972.
4. Powers, Marjorie J.: The unification model in nursing. *Nursing Outlook,* 482–487, August 1976.
5. Sullivan, Judith A.: Comparison of manifest needs of nurses and physicians in primary care practice. *Nursing Research,* 27:255–259, July-August 1978.

4

A Practitioner/Teacher Role for Graduate Program Faculty

Judith Fitzgerald Miller

Faculty members teaching in graduate nursing programs may find themselves far removed from direct patient care and ongoing accountability to patients. Graduate students are primary care givers, in that they follow patients, providing care in many settings—acute hospital, rehabilitation, nursing home, ambulatory care clinics, and at home. Freedom from close faculty surveillance is crucial if the graduate student is to assume successfully the role of graduate clinical practitioner, isolating concepts for study, pursuing answers to research questions, and obtaining specialized nursing competence associated with the advanced practitioner role. Faculty preceptors are aware of the student's case load because they make rounds to meet patients, cursorily assess each patient's health states; review the student's field notes; hold individual conferences with students; and conduct group clinical sessions. Because of the unique needs of graduate students, graduate nursing faculty members are not present on one selected agency unit for several consecutive days a week to observe, plan for, and provide care, as are some faculty members of the undergraduate program. The result may be the graduate program faculty member begins to lose self-confidence and competence in the same practice skills expected from graduate students. The small and unique group of nurses who are doctorally prepared often insulate themselves from clinical practice through teaching, administrative, and research roles. That group of nurses most adequately prepared to generate theories and to provide a scientific foundation for practice often isolate themselves from inductive field research and apply deductive quantitative approaches—a step that may be premature in striving to develop our discipline.

WHY PRACTICE?

The answer to the question, "Why should university faculty members engage in direct nursing practice?" seems obvious when the following questions are analyzed: If faculty members do not have an opportunity to provide care for clients, how can they teach and use examples of patient needs and therapies relevant to today's world? How do faculty members maintain their basic nursing skills and what about their research skills and knowledge of clinical phenomena that need to be investigated? How can a faculty member's sense of inquiry be stimulated so that she can generate research questions that are directly applicable to nursing practice if the faculty member only sets foot in the agency door in a teaching role for students, safely removed from any direct responsibility for patients or accountability to them and their families? How do faculty members make a significant impact on the health care agency so as to improve health care services for the community? How do faculty members advance the science of nursing? Is it merely by studying nursing students, trends, the evolution of the discipline, or by teaching-learning modalities?

To maintain a sense of credibility as a nurse educator with advanced knowledge, the educator must demonstrate a continual progression of insights and knowledge through practice. Maintaining a sense of competence and self-esteem is essential, not only when teaching students but when working with members of related health disciplines. Faculty groups emphasize collaboration and speak of colleagueship. Expectations are set for students to collaborate and relate confidently as a colleague, but what about the faculty member? If the faculty member has no patients in his/her case load to discuss with others, we cannot expect members of related disciplines to respect our knowledge, recognize our abilities, or consult with us in striving to achieve patient outcomes.

I practice professional nursing one half day a week in a diabetic clinic at a medical college center. My graduate students practice in this same medical complex in the inpatient, outpatient, and rehabilitation hospital areas. My reasons for practice include:

- having a current case load of patients to use as examples for teaching my graduate students,
- improving and maintaining clinical expertise with a select group of patients,
- raising research questions and conducting research,
- seeking answers to identified clinical problems through literature review,
- establishing a setting for fellow nursing faculty to utilize for practice,
- demonstrating a practitioner/teacher role to graduate students, university faculty, agency personnel, and medical college faculty.

The focus of my practice is to help patients with expressed needs, mobilizing their self-care assets, developing their self-care abilities, and, in effect, being an advocate for the patient.

NATURE OF THE PRACTICE

There are many avenues through which faculty members can engage in nursing practice roles. A faculty joint appointment with a health care agency and university is one avenue, although this is not feasible or desirable for all faculty members or advanced practitioners within agencies (i.e., primary commitments for curriculum development, ongoing university affairs, and so on, must be managed). (The joint appointment avenue of practice is described elsewhere in this book.) For faculty to make a significant contribution to patient and family care during acute physical crises may demand working a 40-hour week, which is only possible outside the academic calendar (summers or holiday breaks). One realistic avenue for practice that can be managed during the academic year lies in ambulatory care settings. Over a period of time a large case load of patients whose care is managed by the faculty member can be gathered. The time investment may be one or one half day per week.

What are the characteristics of the faculty member's advanced practice? The relationship between practice and research is symbiotic. Everything the practitioner does is typified as systematic, e.g., recording the results of action or observation. The practitioner can use a qualitative research methodology, acting as a participant observer to record data on the phenomena studied. For example, in my work with diabetics I record the self-care practices of the clients I see. I categorize the types of needs ambulatory patients have for professional nursing care. (In this particular agency, hospital administration is questioning the need for nursing care in the outpatient department.) Although my concentrated nursing effort has been with a small case load of patients, I have seen and initiated care plans on 63 patients over the past year. I have also developed an eclectic model for my practice, and tried out the model as well as the assessment tools developed to implement the model.

I believe the essence of nursing in ambulatory settings is to assist individuals to utilize self-care practices to achieve health results. The central focus of nursing may change slightly as individuals move on the health-illness continuum. Figure 4.1 depicts a changing nursing focus as the individual's health state changes from acute illness in phase I to convalescence in phase II and to restored health in phase III.[1]

This model was a result (in part) of my ongoing nursing practice role. I realized that rigid application of one of the proposed nursing frameworks to

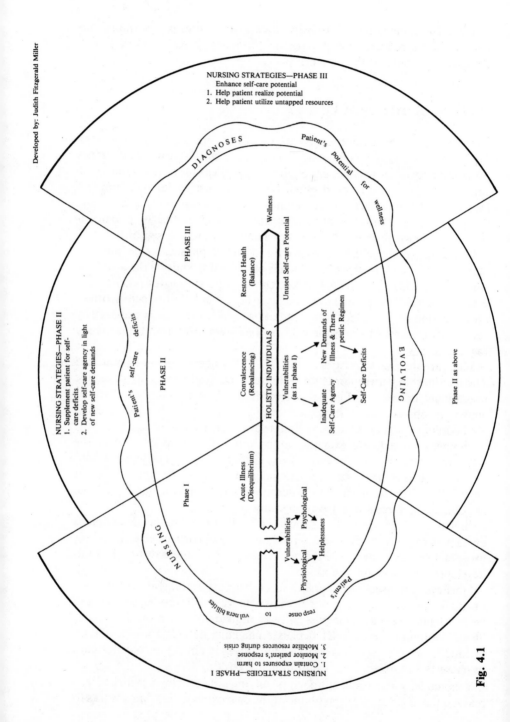

Developed by: Judith Fitzgerald Miller

NURSING STRATEGIES—PHASE III
Enhance self-care potential
1. Help patient realize potential
2. Help patient utilize untapped resources

NURSING STRATEGIES—PHASE II
1. Supplement patient for self-care deficits
2. Develop self-care agency in light of new self-care demands

NURSING STRATEGIES—PHASE I
1. Contain exposures to harm
2. Monitor patient's response
3. Mobilize resources during crisis

DIAGNOSES

Patient's Potential for wellness

PHASE III

PHASE II

Patient's self-care deficits

Phase I

NURSING

EVOLVING

Phase II as above

Patient's response to vulnerabilities

HOLISTIC INDIVIDUALS

Restored Health (Balance) — Wellness
Unused Self-care Potential

Convalescence (Rebalancing)

Vulnerabilities (as in phase I)

New Demands of Illness & Thera- peutic Regimen
Self-Care Deficits

Inadequate Self-Care Agency

Acute Illness (Disequilibrium)

Vulnerabilities
Physiological
Psychological
Helplessness

Fig. 4.1

patients, regardless of their position on the illness-health continuum, may not be appropriate. I believed that my focus on self-care was a viable guide to my practice for my patients in the metabolic clinic, all of whom are in phases II and III of the illness-health continuum. But does a self-care concept provide enough direction for nurses to organize nursing strategies for individuals during acute physiologic and psychological crises? Due to this concern a modified self-care model was developed.

The focus of nursing during phase I includes: (1) containing (halting) exposures to harm; (2) monitoring physiologic and psychosocial responses; and (3) mobilizing patient and family resources during crises. During an acute illness, patient vulnerabilities leading to helplessness may be classified as physiologic and psychosocial. Physiologic vulnerabilities that encompass all medical diagnoses include shock, stress responses, fluid and electrolyte changes, and catabolic changes. Psychosocial vulnerabilities include altered body image, loss, powerlessness, deprivations (sleep, sensory, touch, emotional), role disturbances, and depleted coping resources. As the individual's health state begins to rebalance, the patient enters phase II.[2]

The focus for nursing strategies during phase II includes (1) supplementing the patients due to noted self-care deficits (the individual's inability to maintain health practice) and (2) developing the individual's self-care agency (abilities to initiate and carry out actions to achieve health results) in light of new self-care demands. Self-care demands are a result of an altered health state, prescribed regimen, or patient's desire to reach a higher level of wellness. Examples of some self-care deficits in our ambulatory diabetic patients during phase II are as follows:

- Inability to adhere to a 1200-calorie diet
- Unaware of time and events related to overeating
- Lack of understanding of diabetic exchange lists
- Unable to plan for diet modification when eating out
- Lacks understanding of the fact that his/her obesity, hypertension and uncontrolled diabetes are contributing to vascular disease
- Has not modified salt intake—on Esidrix for hypertension
- Grief over deteriorating physical state despite regimen adherence. Depression over loss of body function
- Unaware of unique strengths and positive coping abilities
- Unexpressed anger and resentment over having diabetes since childhood
- Unable to coordinate therapies for diabetes, arthritis, and hypertension
- Lack of faith in ability to adequately perform roles of mother, wife, and so forth
- Does not exercise

• Injects cold insulin
• Lacks sense of personal worth
• Unsure of expected outcomes of therapy

Phase III is a state of restored health or, for the chronically ill or dying, a state of optimal functioning. During this phase, nursing is centered around enhancing the patient's self-care potential. Helping patients realize their potential and helping them to utilize untapped resources are the nursing challenges.[3]

To examine my practice with patients more explicitly during phase II and III, the following rather straight-forward interpretation of the self-care concept of nursing is presented in Figure 4.2.

This model depicts four major constructs of the self-care concept of practice. Nursing agency overlaps into the areas of self-care agency, therapeutic self-care demands, and self-care deficits because nursing actions are included in all three areas. Nursing is responsible for assessing the individual's self-care action, completing care activities due to the patient's deficits, enhancing the patient's self-care ability, and evaluating the patient's self-care abilities.

The outlined assessment tool (see Table 4.1) for determining the patient's self-care agency is thorough and appropriate for use with hospitalized patients; however, its complete application in initial nursing contacts with ambulatory patients is not feasible. For example, accurate information about the individual's self-concept, locus of control, and role mastery are obtained after a continued helping relationship. It is only possible to complete the data base after a long-term relationship, not after the first outpatient contact with the nurse, which averages 20 minutes. In order to obtain precise information regarding diabetes self-care practices, a specific tool "Self-Care Evaluation for Ambulatory Patients with Diabetes" was devised for each clinic visit (Table 4.2).

Data collected from this self-care evaluation for ambulatory patients with diabetes as well as the assessment of self-care agency tools were analyzed in order to complete care plans on patients coming to the clinic.

With the assistance of a graduate student research assistant, who worked with me in the diabetic clinic for the past semester and summer session, I am recording patient-care outcomes achieved as a result of constant primary professional nursing care in an ambulatory setting over a prolonged period of time. We are in the process of determining these outcomes for a selected number of patients. The outcomes will include an analysis of the patient's clinical and behavioral status before and after long-term professional nursing care. The clinical outcomes refer to physiologic parameters—blood

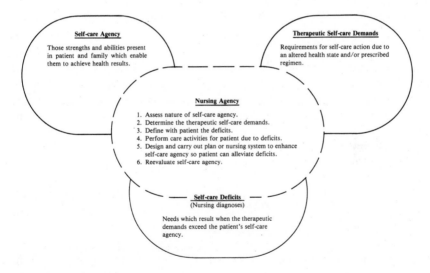

Self-care Agency

Those strengths and abilities present in patient and family which enable them to achieve health results.

Therapeutic Self-care Demands

Requirements for self-care action due to an altered health state and/or prescribed regimen.

Nursing Agency

1. Assess nature of self-care agency.
2. Determine the therapeutic self-care demands.
3. Define with patient the deficits.
4. Perform care activities for patient due to deficits.
5. Design and carry out plan or nursing system to enhance self-care agency so patient can alleviate deficits.
6. Reevaluate self-care agency.

Self-care Deficits
(Nursing diagnoses)

Needs which result when the therapeutic demands exceed the patient's self-care agency.

Fig. 4.2. Self-Care Model. Developed by Judith Fitzgerald Miller from Orem, Dorothea: Nursing: Concepts of Practice. New York: McGraw-Hill, 1971 and Nursing Development Conference Group: Concept Formalization in Nursing. Boston, Little, Brown, & Co., 1973.

Table 4.1   Assessment Guide For Self-Care Agency

The following categories of information need to be analyzed in order to make definitive decisions about the adequacy of a patient's self-care agency:

A.   Growth and development state of the individual

B.   Individual's self-concept. Self-concept is the most important factor affecting human behavior—
—Body image
—Personal self, i.e., self-ideal, self-expectations, values, moral self, self-consistency
—Self-esteem
What is the reference from which the individual makes decisions regarding his health state?
At what point in the development of symptoms do these changes have meaning? Or are regarded as significant by the patient?
When does the individual value taking action regarding these symptoms?
(The individual's feelings of worth, esteem or lack of these affect the initiation of deliberate action to achieve a better health state.)
—Perceived locus of control—internal or external

C.   Health state—physical and mental state
—Body system review to determine functional ability
—Mental status
—Consider the therapeutic self-care demands placed upon the individual due to illness state, prescribed regimen. These may be listed as therapeutic self-care demands with resulting self-care deficits defined.

D.   Routine health care practices
—Habits
—Diet
—Exercise
—Avoidance of allergens, environmental hazards
—Use of leisure time
—Universal self-care needs—how met
Air, food, water, elimination, activity-rest, solitude-social interaction, planning for a sense of normalcy

E.   Level of motivation
—May be impaired due to factors other than physical health changes or fatigue; may be due to lack of readiness, phase of adjustment to the chronic health problem, psychological immobilization

—Ability to determine goals, take action to achieve an end
—Attitude toward body may affect, e.g., testing urine

F. Level of understanding
    —Capacity for learning
    —Attention span
    —Ability to grasp new ideas, concepts
    —Attitude toward new self-care behaviors
    —Readiness to incorporate new knowledge into repertoire of behaviors
    —Scientifically derived knowledge about self-care in terms of disorders present
    —Source of present information

G. Place in the family constellation
    —Role of significant others
    —Support network present

H. Resources
    —What resources for continuing development of self-care agency are available
     to the patient?
    —Is patient capable of seeking out and utilizing the resources?

I. Problem-solving ability

J. Previous coping style

K. Personal factors
    —Occupation, economic status
    —Living alone or with others who can participate in care
    —Role of faith, religion
    —Membership in groups other than the family
    —Culture
    —Meaning of this illness

L. Role mastery
    —Role conflict present
    —Phase of role transition

M. Life-change units experienced within past 6 months to 1 year

N. Other unique strengths of this individual

Table 4.2 Self-Care Evaluation for Ambulatory Patients with Diabetes

I.   Interview

    A.   Diet
       Calorie restriction
       Exchange list knowledge
       Problems, dietary indiscretion
       Weight control
       Actual Weight_____Ideal Weight_____
       Diet history
          Foods important to life style
          Usual daily meal pattern (write on back of page)

    B.   Insulin
       Site rotation
       Storage of

    C.   Exercise
       Type
       Frequency

    D.   Urine Testing
       Method Used_____Where stored_____
       Results _____ Record kept _____
       Action taken when over 1% and ketones present

    E.   Hypoglycemic reactions
       Pattern (time and related events)
       Frequency
       Action taken

    F.   Patient needs in coming to clinic today

    G.   Adjustment to diabetes
       How does diabetes affect life style?
       Impact on family

    H.   Activities that enhance or maintain self-esteem

    I.   Other health problems and medication regimen

II.   Physical

    A.   B.P.
    B.   Circulation
       Skin
       Pulses
    C.   Feet
       Pressure points

Routine foot care, nails, cleanliness
Appropriate shoes
Calluses, corns
D. Gums
E. Vision changes
F. Neuropathy

III. Nurse's interpretation of findings

Overall compliance
Evaluation of patient's emotional state
Patient's ability to grasp new concepts—capacity for learning

IV. Mutually determined goals

---

sugar, urine sugar and ketones, and weight. Behavioral outcomes refer to role changes; psychological states of affect and self-esteem; adherence to regimens; and self-care practices.

To maintain a research focus does not require the nurse to design an experimental or quasiexperimental approach. It does mean that the nurse systematically examines, in a phenomenologic manner, a problem or isolated concept, e.g., the patient's coping style or strategies, the meaning of illness in obesity, powerlessness, social isolation in chronic illness, help-seeking behavior, mechanisms that enhance self-esteem, and life events related to the diagnoses of illness. Documenting the individual's responses to care over a period of time, recording patient-reported early symptoms of hypoglycemia, or documenting role transition and evaluating efforts of role supplementation are other examples of research.

The impetus for one of my current research efforts stemmed from my clinic practice role. In working with black patients, I was impressed repeatedly with our interactions in that the blacks, especially males, seemed to be very controlled in their verbal and nonverbal responses; showing little facial expression, not altering voice volume or pitch, and not using affective vocalizations. Black patients for the most part avoided eye contact when they were talking to me (a white nurse); they seldom initiated discussions. Due to these observations, I began to wonder how black patients communicated to nurses when they were in acute need, for example, their need for pain relief. I collaborated with a professor in interpersonal communications from the college of speech at our university to design the communications study, "Pain Expression Styles of Individuals from Different Cultures." We studied 60 subjects (24 black and 36 white) who were experiencing pain to determine their verbal and nonverbal pain-expression behaviors. Process recordings of four-minute interviews are being analyzed to determine pain-disclosure patterns and free discussions of pain-relief therapy. A nonverbal pain behavior scale was also completed after each interview and validated by two data collectors, both nurses. The results of this study should help nurses to become sensitive to the communication styles of individuals from different cultures.

My nursing practice in the clinic is being observed by the staff, other health professionals, and students. Graduate students come to the diabetic clinic to observe me and to work with me. I collaborate with graduate students about nursing care decisions. I also receive feedback about prescribed nursing strategies from nurse practitioners with master's degrees who are working with diabetics in the agency as well as from graduate students.

The practice is characterized by its responsibility for managing the nursing care of a case load of patients. I am accountable to the patients and their families as well as to the nurse practitioner employed in the diabetes clinic. I collaborate with the medical staff of endocrinology.

One of the reasons for investing time and effort in practicing professional nursing in this clinic is to demonstrate a professional nursing role to the medical college physician faculty who provide medical care in the clinic. In some instances physicians hold nurses in high esteem, if the nurse systematically organizes the charts, carefully files the lab slips, follows delegated orders precisely and efficiently, and does not slow up the progress of M.D.s who are examining a quota number of patients in a set clinic time. Nurses in this situation can easily become advocates for the physician's work instead of realizing they have a unique role of their own to play, helping patients with expressed needs, mobilizing the patient's self-care assets, developing their self-care abilities, and, in effect, being advocates for the patient. Most physicians have yet to see the results of working together (nurse, physician, and patient) to achieve patient outcomes. Physician contact with any nurses prepared beyond a baccalaureate level is limited. One of my concerns was to change the physician's concept of the nurse's role, improving nursing's image so that we could work together to help the patients achieve health results. An even greater concern was that a nurse's potential for services to patients was untapped. A better health state would result if patients had the opportunity to be in contact with a professional nurse in addition to the M.D. All of my efforts to establish collegial relationships facilitated the graduate students' collaboration with physicians regarding patients.

IMPACT ON DEVELOPING NURSING'S KNOWLEDGE BASE

The university's mission is to discover knowledge and disseminate it. Nursing faculty members are challenged with this responsibility. However, only recently have nurse researchers begun to focus on clinical nursing studies in which research is desperately needed to shape the practice of nursing. Fewer studies of nurses, the nursing profession, and teaching are being undertaken. Without clinical research, the substantive content of the discipline will not develop.

University faculty members, by the very nature of their roles and standards for their evaluation, must keep abreast of research in their specialty areas. When working directly with patients and staff, they have an opportunity to help the staff and the patients (when appropriate) become aware of latest research findings. Thus, the well-known gap between research findings and implementation can be narrowed. Faculty members will have submerged themselves in a wide range of literature (research from supporting disciplines as well as nursing) and will be able to share vast amounts of knowledge.

Research is not reserved for a group of academic elite securely housed in university offices, safe from confronting patient problems or from providing therapeutic services to patients for students and all to scrutinize. Research need not be a sterile, rigid, esoteric endeavor.

Medicine arrived at theories for practice by keeping clinical journals, i.e., recording patient symptoms, prescribed interventions, and the results of therapy. Nurses who practice with patients need to keep clinical field notes of patients in their case loads. These notes should contain strategies and outcomes. Systematic refinement of the framework that guides practice is also needed and could be kept in journals. Faculty members need to pioneer in developing our discipline by engaging in *clinical* research. Ours is a practice discipline, lacking a scientific base.

Investigators need to develop research tools that are appropriate devices for research in nursing. At times, we have inappropriately borrowed tools without modification from psychology or other disciplines, which may or may not have been appropriate for nursing. Devising procedures and tools results from direct clinical observations and involvement.

According to Chin and Jacobs, concept analysis is the first of a four-staged process of theory development.[4] (The other three stages are formulating and testing related statements, writing the theory, and applying the theory.) Making decisions about selecting relevant concepts that need to be thoroughly examined takes place in the clinical setting. After the concepts are selected, literature on them must be thoroughly reviewed. What appeared to be simplistic and well understood, is now more complex, and more implications for patient care have been generated. The concept to be studied is discovered in the clinical setting, and a descriptive or qualitative method is used. It can be seen that the first stage of theory development calls for the rigorous, clinical participation of the faculty member.

A dearth of theories underlie nursing practice. However, concepts describing and categorizing facts (exploratory theory building) need to be isolated. Using an inductive approach means to immerse the researcher in a world of subjects. Studying phenomena from the subject's point of view is a preliminary step in the development of nursing theory.

The process of initiating the faculty practice role has been very challenging. Initially, nursing administration hesitated about providing me with practice privileges, and the fact that my graduate students were able to provide care to clients, enjoying unrestricted care privileges in this setting, whereas I was not, was indeed perplexing. It took some patience and understanding on my part to allow time for nursing service administration to adjust to the idea of an advanced practitioner working with clients in their agency without receiving monetary compensation. An understandable expressed concern was legal accountability for a professional who was not employed by the agency. However, I carry individual malpractice insurance. When the hospital administration was informed of my request for practice privileges, my practice role was sanctioned without hesitation.

It was apparent that efforts devoted to developing interpersonal relationships with the agency staff (nurses, clerks, aides, as well as physicians) would determine the success or failure of the practitioner/teacher's role in the clinic. Agency nurses were suspicious of my work. But, this lack of trust was overcome by long-term practice in the setting, by conferring with them about clients, and by having them interpret agency policy.

I was also successful in having the position for a master's prepared nurse established to provide continuous professional care for clinic patients, because the agency provides clinics for patients with diabetes three days a week. Programs for patients, protocols for patient teaching, and consultation with nursing staff for inpatient care needed to be designed and implemented. To obtain support for this position, as in meeting other challenges, I aligned myself with the medical college physician faculty, who wielded the power within the organization. Having demonstrated the potential role of an advanced practitioner, the medical staff, together with nursing service, presented a proposal to the hospital administration for the position, which was approved and funded.

TEACHING RESPONSIBILITIES

Although my faculty responsibilities include teaching all or part of other course content, some to undergraduates, my principal role function as teacher of graduate students is through the seminar-practicum course, Nursing Strategies for Adults: Long Term Health Problems, the content of which is mutually reinforcing for my practice. Graduate students enrolled in this course practice in the same medical complex in which I provide care to ambulatory patients with diabetes. This four-credit graduate clinical nursing course is the first of a two-course sequence designed to develop the student's advanced practice skills. The course builds upon the student's knowledge obtained in the core courses: Theories of Nursing, Role Development, and Dynamics of Behavior and Nursing Intervention. In my clinic practice I am able to demonstrate concepts emphasized in these core courses, i.e., operationalizing a nursing conceptual framework, role appropriation, and family counseling, respectively, to students. I am also able to demonstrate a way to achieve the objectives of this practicum course.

The nursing strategies course is designed to help students analyze the physiologic and psychosocial responses as well as the coping mechanisms of individuals with long-term health problems.The students provide care to a case load of patients (and families) for one academic semester. The case load is defined by the student's special interests, and throughout the program efforts are made to help the student develop expertise with this type of patient or patient problem. In this course, students are introduced to a qualitative research methodology, an approach that characterizes their nursing practice. Field notes are kept throughout the semester on observations recorded on an isolated concept being studied in depth. The field notes also document use of a nursing conceptual framework, application of research findings, suggestions for research studies, and a host of other data (Table 4.3). This exercise satisfies many objectives and hopefully piques the student's sense of inquiry.

The coping tasks of the chronically ill make up the seminar topics of the course. The typology of coping tasks was arrived at through joint study by graduate students and myself.[5]

A variety of learning experiences are designed to help students achieve the course objectives. The objectives are designed to expand the students' knowledge of concepts related to the chronically ill, to enhance their skills in caring for select client groups, to operationalize a conceptual framework for nursing, to incorporate qualitative research into daily nursing practice, and to use a qualitative methodology to study an isolated clinical concept as an initial phase in micro or middle-range theory development.

Although it is beyond the scope of this chapter to describe all details and learning experiences of this course, one aspect, the efforts of students and faculty mutually pursuing answers to research questions, relates to the purposes of this book.

Table 4.3   Guide for Writing Field Notes

The purpose in writing field notes is to help the graduate student begin qualitative data collection. In recording data, the student will have the opportunity to analyze: the patient's response to his health problem, the nursing care administered, and outcomes of care.

Specific types of data which may be recorded in the field notes include:

Patient profiles
Physiologic and psychosocial behavior
Prescribed medical therapies which affect nursing
Nursing diagnoses
Nursing care given
Outcomes of nursing care
Impact of conceptual framework on nursing practice
Documentation from literature which enhanced understanding
Research questions generated from observations and practice
New insights—application of seminar content
                critical indicators of existing nursing diagnoses
                new nursing diagnoses
Impact of the chronic illness on:
   daily activities—leisure, work
   family interaction
   role disturbance
   self-esteem
   emerging coping patterns
   self-care abilities
   help seeking behavior—assigning meaning to symptoms
   grief work
   social isolation
Evaluation of student's contribution

The field notes must include:
1. Patient profile
2. Student documentation on the student's selected clinical focus or clinical concept, e.g., powerlessness, altered energy, coping strategies
3. Demonstration of the use of a conceptual framework for nursing
4. Posing research questions

I have already referred to a symbiotic relationship between practice and research. This relationship also exists between teaching, practice, and research (see Fig. 4.3). The faculty member is functioning to his/her fullest capacity when the symbiotic relationship can be demonstrated. Williamson raises questions about faculty members becoming more professor than practitioner.[6] In a practice discipline, this should not be possible; the practitioner-teacher-researcher role components for university nursing faculty members are inseparable. There is a cyclic effect on one role component due to the others.

A tool called The Impact of Chronic Illness was designed to help students gain insights into the world of the chronically ill as well as contribute to a data pool about the chronically ill (see Table 4.4). Categories of insights for the graduate student include the patient's social isolation, self-esteem, symptom-control activities, grief/work coping styles and strategies, and nursing diagnoses. For the past seven academic semesters, 71 graduate students who completed this course have collected data on the 198 patients comprising their case loads. Because the tool was revised, data from the first semester in which it was used will not be included in the final analysis. Data from 187 chronically ill subjects (collected by 65 graduate students) are being analyzed to answer the following research questions about self-esteem:

1. What are specific indicators of high or low self-esteem observed by professional nurses in chronically ill individuals?
2. What are specific indicators of high or low self-esteem reported by chronically ill individuals?
3. What is the relationship between the patient's self-report of feelings of worth and the nurse's interpretation of the patient's self-esteem?
4. What is the relationship between positive self-esteem and the presence of significant others as a support system to the chronically ill individual?
5. Is there a relationship between time lapse since the diagnosis of a chronic illness and self-esteem?
6. Is there a relationship between the number of exacerbations of the illness and patient reported self-esteem?
7. Do individuals with a chronic illness selectively engage in activities to enhance their self-esteem?
8. Is there a relationship between an individual's help-seeking and level of self-esteem?

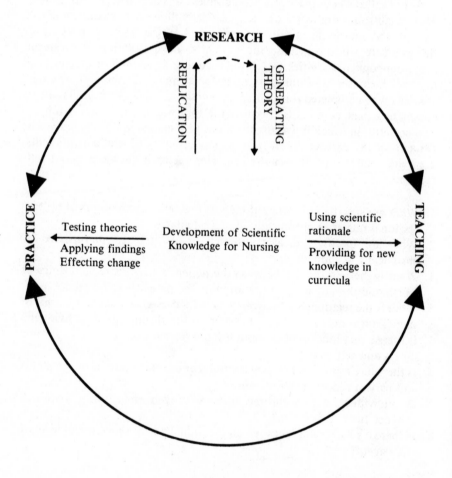

Fig. 4.3.   Symbiotic relationship of practice, teaching, and research for university faculty members.

Table 4.4   Impact of Chronic Illness

Student's   Name _____

Today's   Date _____

Patient's   age _____

Patient's   sex _____

Medical diagnosis _____ Date first diagnosed _____

Number of exacerbations of this health problem _____

Marital status _____ Children, ages _____

Social Isolation

Family Interaction
1. What role do the significant others play in the patient's life adjustment? (e.g., assist with care regime; loving support system, etc.) List the person, their specific activities, and whether they live with the patient.

2. Does the patient have someone to talk with each day? If yes, list relationship.

Stage in Life Career
1. Describe work role, i.e., occupation, years at this type work, currently working.

2. Have symptoms progressed to interfere with work or do symptoms prevent continuing employment?

Role Count
1. List roles which have been eliminated as a result of the chronic health problem.

2. Summarize what roles the individual continues to play.

3. What leisure activities does the patient engage in?

4. What social activities have had to be eliminated?

Key Nursing Diagnoses (Please feel free to digress from the established typology.)

Nurse Observed Indicators of Self-Esteem

Describe indicators of your patient's high or low self-esteem which you have observed. (Refer to the self-esteem indicators guide). Also review behaviors you have documented in your field notes which indicate this patient's feelings of worth or worthlessness.

Low   **High**

Patient-Reported Indicators of Self-Esteem (record verbatim responses)
1. Has having _____ changed how you feel about yourself?
                                    (diagnosis)
   (If so, in what way?)

2. Describe your attitude toward yourself.

3. In evaluating your abilities, how would you describe yourself?

4. Do you have a positive or negative attitude toward yourself?

5. What do you do to feel good about yourself?
   (Describe the activities the patient selectively engages in to achieve a sense of success, accomplishment, to enhance self-esteem.)

Symptom Control

1. What prompts this patient to seek medical-nursing attention?

2. What are indicators of powerlessness manifested by this patient?

3. What is the relationship between patient's perceived powerlessness and his help-seeking behavior?

Grieving over Losses

1. Summarize the losses the patient has suffered since the onset of his/her chronic illness.

Coping

1. What coping style does the patient tend to prefer?

2. Describe the coping strategies this patient utilizes which lead to your conclusion regarding coping style. (Summarize from your field notes.)

3. Does the patient use any technique adjunctive to the prescribed therapy? (e.g., TM, meditation, mind control, relaxation exercises, etc.)

4. Include any other pertinent data you feel would be helpful in understanding this patient's coping with the health problem.

Patient's name _____

Patient's address _____

Patient's phone _____

Patient needs future contacts from other graduate

students _____

Patient has been consulted about future contacts by

graduate students _____

Specific sections of data from the Impact of Chronic Illness inventory have been analyzed and will be reported in Judith Miller's book *Coping With Powerlessness of Chronic Illness* (1981). Findings from the data on coping have been categorized into types of coping tasks of the chronically ill. Exhaustive lists of coping strategies utilized by patients on either end of a coping continuum (approach or avoidance) were compiled. The results of the research have helped to reshape this practitioner course.

Data collected on the Impact of Chronic Illness inventory resulted from a primary care giver's long-term knowledge of the patient. Data of this nature could not be collected on large numbers of patients by an isolated researcher.

IMPACT OF PRACTITIONER/TEACHER ROLE

The effect my practitioner/teacher role has had on students and other faculty has been noted. I have been able to demonstrate advanced practice to graduate students enrolled in my course Nursing Strategies for Adults: Long-Term Health Problems. Graduate students have been able to work with a case load of clients from the clinic. Research ideas have been developed in collaboration with graduate students. Data collection by some students for their master's program research project has begun in this practicum course. Graduate students can see for themselves a faculty member's successes and failures in achieving patient outcomes. Interchange about real world clinical problems with students challenge and inspire them to reach and set new standards of practice.

The present and potential impact of this role is impressive. The faculty practice role has been contagious, in that two faculty colleagues developed similar practices suited to their specialty areas, oncology and respiratory care. One faculty member spent her sabbatical leave studying and caring for patients in the diabetes clinic and in an oncology clinic; a nursing doctoral student's clinical practicum took place in the diabetes clinic. These experiences were made possible because of my efforts, over a one-year time-span, in developing the practitioner/teacher role in this setting.

This effort would not have taken place without the release-time provided by H.E.W. Grant 5 D23 NU000 38-03 entitled Expanding a Role-Oriented Model for Graduate Education. However, now that the ground work has been completed, it is possible for me to continue my clinic activities one morning a week, with a full-time teaching load. My voluntary clinic work continues over the summer, when the graduate program is not in session.

University expectations and evaluation procedures for faculty in schools of nursing have made some nurse educators become so eager to be "part of the university" that they have taken on behaviors of faculty in nonpractice disciplines: relegating a practice role to have low status, consuming time from "pure" theory construction. In our struggle to become a scholarly discipline, have we forgotten that we are also a professional discipline with a commitment to practice?

REFERENCES

1. Miller, Judith F.: The dynamic focus of nursing: A challenge to nursing administration. *The Journal of Nursing Administration,* 10:13–18, 1980.
2. Ibid.
3. Ibid.
4. Chin, Peggy and Jacobs, Maeona: A model for theory development in nursing. *Advances in Nursing Science,* 1:1–11, October 1978.
5. Miller, Judith F.: *Coping with Powerlessness of Chronic Illness.* Philadelphia, F.A. Davis, Probable Publication Date, 1981.
6. Williamson, Janet: More professor than practitioner? In Williamson, Janet (ed.): *Current Perspectives in Nursing Education: The Changing Scene.* St. Louis, C.V. Mosby Co., 1976, pp. 80–85.

II
The Academic Side of the Role

Introduction

Lorraine Machan

Colleges of nursing still lag far behind in providing an atmosphere for full academic development.[1] Even in those institutions fortunate enough to have acquired research-oriented faculty members, these are, for the large part, the exception; research is left to the small minority while the majority find readily available excuses.

Perhaps the greatest detriment to professional nursing is the doctorally prepared faculty member who has no therapeutic function and no research function. Enjoying the security of her tenure and the status of her title, for her the nature of the doctoral degree is indeed "terminal," signifying the end of scholarly effort. Unfortunately many neophyte faculty members have been socialized into the concept of academic role provided by her example. Until and unless the faculty in colleges of nursing demonstrate that practice, teaching, and research can be combined into one role, nursing has no legitimate claim as an academic professional discipline. Unless doctorally prepared nurses can demonstrate that the doctoral degree enables them to practice nursing in a way that really improves the quality of care given and in a way that differs from the nurse without a doctorate, then there is no legitimate reason, from the standpoint of the profession as a whole, for nurses to obtain doctoral degrees.

Joanne Stevenson (Ch. 7) points out that the "pervading concept of a nurse is almost an antithesis to the traditional image of the researcher." Nursing as a profession has made considerable progress in establishing its identity as a profession. It has not as yet made much progress in identifying what the nature of its research should be. Accepting research as part of practice might be less of a problem if nurse researchers made less use of traditional methods designed for and by other disciplines and tried approaches more in keeping with the nature of nursing.[2]

In their provocative paper, Reconsidering the Relation Between Theory/ Research and Practice, Buckholdt and Gubrium (1976) state: "Practitioners in or about academe may suffer the pride of a minority group: a devalued conception of their ability to deal adequately with how to put theory and research to work." Although the paper is speaking about the discipline of sociology, the description of the "conventional boundary between theory/ research and practice" is equally applicable to the discipline of nursing.[3]

The practitioner/teacher who accepts a University appointment faces one of the most exciting challenges nursing has to offer. She not only can change the way nursing is practiced, she can change the way nursing is taught.

Discussing faculty role development in university nursing programs, Barley and Redman conceptualized the continuum of development to a full faculty role as passing from "single role awareness" as teachers to "full role functioning" with the ability to "move easily within several roles frequently and simultaneously."[4] These same authors point out that because of the rapid changes taking place in the field of nursing, adaptation to these changes necessitates ongoing change and development not only in the individual but in the institution. Just as Basteyns (Ch. 2) described how an understanding nursing administrator made it possible for her to function differently from other nurses, so too must deans of nursing colleges encourage and promote a change in the interpretation of the faculty role. Whereas we now find few faculty members in colleges of nursing who really combine practice, teaching, and research, the picture should be just the opposite. There should be very few, if any, who do not practice the discipline they are teaching, with research as an inherent part of that practice.

In Chapter 5 Helen Harrington traces historic trends in the profession that have led to the dilemma in which many nurse educators find themselves. One answer to her suggestion that perhaps efforts should be put into upgrading professional practitioners rather than expecting the faculty member to take on a practice role is well expressed by Marjorie Powers:

> Indeed it is not likely that we will get anywhere in changing organizational approaches in nursing at the university level if we continue to wait for the so-called critical mass of change agents (clinicians) to emerge. . . . The only alternative is to broaden the expectations for nursing faculty to include managment of patient care as well as the investigation of clinical problems.[5]

The chapter by Mary Conway and Laurie Glass describes problems en-countered by neophyte faculty members and the importance of planned socialization to an academic role. The authors offer insight that is not only valuable to faculty members developing an academic role, but also provides a viewpoint that can be valuable to nursing deans in their efforts to convince university administrators that practice disciplines cannot be placed in a tenure framework designed for nonpractice disciplines.

The chapters by Joanne Stevenson provide a model for developing and strengthening research skills. The model is applicable to either practice or university settings.

The practitioner/teacher, above all others, is in a key position to speed the slowly developing momentum of nursing research. Receiving her stimulus to carry out research from the university community, she should be able to bring enthusiasm for and understanding of the need to see research *as an inherent part of her practice.*

REFERENCES

1. Machan, Lorraine: The obligation of nursing as an academic discipline to preserve liberal education. *Nursing Forum*, Vol. 16:No. 2, 1977.
2. Donaldson, Sue K. and Crowley, Dorothy M.: The discipline of nursing. *Nursing Outlook,* 26:113–120, Feb. 1978.
3. Buckholdt, David R. and Gubrium, Jaber F.: Reconsidering the relation between theory/research and practice. *Sociological Practice*, 1:105–115, Fall 1976.
4. Barley, Zoe A. and Redman, Barbara K.: Faculty role development in university schools of nursing. *Journal of Nursing Administration*, 9:43–47, May 1979.
5. Powers, Marjorie: The unification model in nursing. *Nursing Outlook*, 24:482–487, August 1976.

5

The Nurse Educator's Dilemma

Helen Harrington

Higher education is a characteristic feature of American life. Post-secondary education is no longer reserved for aspiring physicians, lawyers, and clergy. Rather, colleges and universities are accepted as legitimate training grounds for prospective members of the newer professions and occupations.

Throughout the history of higher education, the university professor has been accorded status and prestige. He has been given the role of scholar, committed to generating new knowledge and to assisting students to discover and use what is known. Because his contribution to society has been recognized as essential, his job-related responsibilities have been designed to enhance his ability to perform both facets of his role. It is recognized that blocks of time for reflection, reading, and critical thinking are absolutely essential if research ideas are to be generated, nurtured, and carried to fruition. Therefore, student contact-hours per week have been closely monitored and controlled, school vacation periods have been free of meetings, and sabbatical leave programs have been established.

Nursing is one of the newer disciplines on the higher education scene. The first university-controlled program of nursing was established at the University of Minnesota in 1909. Although this was a milestone for nursing, it was only the beginning of a long struggle to have nursing recognized as a legitimate scholarly discipline deserving of equality and autonomy within the system of higher education. The move to establish baccalaureate education as the basic preparation for professional practice has gained greater acceptance as each year passes. However, although nursing has been accepted as an authentic discipline and nurse faculty members have been accorded rank and other rights bestowed on university faculty, they have not characteristically assumed all of the duties of the role. "Nursing education has won admission to academe but, for full acceptance its professors must meet the same expectations for scholarly productivity, especially with respect to research and publications, as their colleagues in other disciplines."[1]

Several factors contribute to the present status of nurse educators. At a time when many highly qualified, doctorally prepared persons in other disciplines are unable to secure university positions, nursing programs are unable to fill all of their budgeted positions. In baccalaureate and higher degree programs in the United States, 555 budgeted positions were unfilled in 1978.[2] In addition, the positions occupied were most often filled with persons whose academic preparations were less than those of their peers in other disciplines. The educational preparation of faculty in baccalaureate and higher degree programs nationally in 1978 was as follows: 11.9 percent were doctorally prepared, 81.1 percent had master's preparation, and 7 percent held a baccalaureate degree only.[3] By virtue of their preparation, the majority of these faculty members are ill-equipped to meet the level of scholarship expected of a university faculty member.

A second factor of major importance to consider is the inability of most nurse faculty members to arrange blocks of time for reflection and study, critical to generating research ideas and to research-based teaching. Unfilled budgeted positions are but one cause of the problem.

An educational program preparing a professional practitioner demands a great deal of communication and mutual planning among faculty if objectives are to be met. This often results in more meetings and planning sessions than are necessary in most other disciplines. In addition, because nursing is a practice discipline, practicum courses are essential. Nurse faculty members most frequently find their student contact hours are approximately triple those of their peers from other disciplines. Granted, there are other professional programs within the university, but these who have achieved full university status have been a part of the system for many years. As Barrett stated: "Physicians, lawyers, and clergy have held faculty posts in major universities since before the ninth century. In that sense, they have had 11 centuries to work out both a *modus operandi* and a *modus vivendi*, with the sometimes competing requirements of professional practice and faculty status."[4]

Perhaps less compelling, but nevertheless historically documented, nurses themselves are often antischolarly. Many see little need for expanding their knowledge base or formulating a conceptual framework for practice. Rather, they are concerned with the technologic skills of nursing and expend their energies in enhancing their abilities in this area exclusively.[5]

Despite the barriers enumerated above, we currently find increasing numbers of nurse faculty members establishing themselves as full-fledged university professors. However, as we are just beginning to see the development of theory, increased research productivity, and research-based teaching among nurse faculty members, a new concern looms on the horizon; a concern which, if not handled astutely, can disrupt the positive changes taking place.

For the past 8 to 10 years, increasing emphasis has been placed on clinical competence in postbaccalaureate education. This can readily be noted by contrasting today's master's and doctoral programs with those of a decade ago. Programs emphasizing the functional preparation of a teacher or administrator have been replaced by ones that prepare advanced nurse practitioners and clinical specialists. This trend is to be lauded. Clinical competence is most certainly a requisite for any practice discipline. However, this trend has, in my mind, created a dilemma for the nurse educator, a dilemma that is not easily resolved.

At a time when the nurse-teacher is finally gaining some credibility as a university faculty member, she is being forced to either apologize for her lack of recent "hands-on patient care" or to find time amid her other duties to carry a client case load. The rationale given by those who believe nurse educators should also be practitioners include some of the following arguments: you cannot teach what you do not practice; authentic case material is necessary to help students learn emerges from practice; teacher credibility is diminished when the teacher is not viewed as a role model. Compelling as these arguments are, they can, when taken at face value, lead us away from what we wish to accomplish. There is much similarity between expecting a university professor to assume the role of teacher and practitioner and the situation nursing found itself in 20 years ago. At that time nurses often found themselves assuming duties recognized as those of physicians, pharmacists, dietitians, or therapists when these persons were not present. Little thought was given to strategies designed to facilitate the proper allocation of responsibilities. Rather, in the name of good patient care, nurses found themselves doctoring for the doctor when he was not available and helping the patient with activities and exercises within the domain of other therapists when the department was closed for the day or for weekends. Expecting nurses to assume roles other than their own worked to the detriment of the nursing care patients deserved. Today, nurse faculty members are being asked to assume the role of practitioner and teacher. Few attempts are directed toward identifying ways in which the nurse faculty member and nurse practitioner can work together, each assuming their own roles, to strengthen the profession as a whole.

Our credibility as teachers depends not so much on what we do when we are away from students but what we do while we are working with them.

Given the educational preparation of most faculty members today with advanced preparation in practice, it can be argued that they are clinically competent. This competence can be maintained and enhanced as they work with their students in practicum courses. While assisting students to operate within a nursing framework, to use the nursing process to identify and meet patient needs, and to establish productive relationships, the faculty members' skills are continually being tested and refined. In a very real sense, the instructor is role-modeling the intellectual and often technical operations essential to professional practice. Role-modeling the practitioner role, with all that it implies, must be the function of the practitioner. We have all heard the old refrain, "But we have no good role models." Perhaps our energies should be directed to upgrading the professional practitioner, the person responsible and accountable for patient care, rather than placing an additional burden on the faculty member who has a full-time position.

Assuming responsibility for the nursing needs of a case load of clients is time consuming. The legitimate focus must be on the client and his needs, not on the needs of the care giver for authentic case data or skill acquisition. All of us who have assumed this role of care giver realize it is present oriented, unpredictable in terms of intensity of need, and emotionally as well as physically draining.

I submit we do ourselves and our profession a disservice when we expect one person to assume two roles, each of which is legitimate, provides an essential service, requires continual study and skill refinement, and deserves total professional immersion. Rather we must recognize that faculty members need time to execute the responsibilities they are held accountable for which are helping students prepare for professional practice and advancing nursing through research and publication. The time they have must be spent refining their skills as educators (facilitators of learning and providers of substantive content), developing their research skills, and improving their publication records. As they work with students in the practice setting, they should be able to maintain their clinical competence, obtain authentic clinical case material, and role-model professional behaviors.

However, given an organizational structure like the one presented by Christman in part one of this book, the practitioner-teacher role has a high probability of success. The organizational format is designed to reduce role ambiguity and safeguard against role deprivation. In an environment that allows full expression of the practitioner/teacher role, the wedding of the practitioner and the teacher role could prove to be the solution to many of our problems today. Without that environment, however, it is disruptive to increase the nurse faculty member's insecurities or to make her feel like a second-class citizen in her chosen profession because she is incapable of assuming responsibility for two full-time positions.

REFERENCES

1. Arminger, Sister Bernadette. Scholarship in nursing. *Nursing Outlook*, 22:160-164, March 1974.
2. National League for Nursing—NLN Nursing Data Book. National League for Nursing, New York, 1978.
3. Ibid.
4. Barrett, Evelyn R. Academic Nurse Educators: Mobility versus Stability. In Williamson, Janet (ed.): *Current Perspectives in Nursing Education: The Changing Scene.* Vol. 2. St. Louis, C.V. Mosby, 1978.
5. Ibid.

6

Socialization for Survival in the Academic World

Mary E. Conway and Laurie K. Glass

Success in academia for nurse faculty members may at best be accidental and at worst be the outcome of an arduous struggle to interpret conflicting norms and to survive early and unexpected derailment from the tenure track. The disparity between the ideal and the real is often great, and nursing's traditional model for socialization into the academic world may actually impede rather than foster a successful outcome.

While the university has long been regarded as a privileged work place, with the title "professor" conjuring up the image of a scholarly pedant sitting in a booklined office conversing pleasantly with a student, or standing in front of a room full of intent listeners and discoursing on a subject on which he is an acknowledged authority, the actuality is a little different. Thus, the professor today must be aware of a certain amount of public skepticism and distrust about higher education in general. He is likely to be less revered than questioned.

The impact of mediated learning, the spectre of a "teacherless" campus, and students' increasing insistence on having a say in the teaching-learning process create additional anxieties for the teacher. Finally, there is the realization that the total number of faculty openings in the traditional disciplines is shrinking and that as departments become filled with tenured faculty there will be even less room for young graduates attempting to enter the ranks of academia.

The situation with respect to nursing is quite different, however. Fewer than one-third of faculty presently teaching in university schools of nursing are prepared at the requisite level, and relatively fewer of those in rank are tenured, as compared with academics in other disciplines.[1] Thus, there is room for younger nurse scholars who wish to make their careers in the academic world. Whether they will actually achieve successful careers, however, will depend a great deal on their introduction and socialization into that world. As one young faculty member expressed it, "The school of nursing is like a sorority, where the junior faculty are put through an extended 'Hell Week,' killing themselves as they seek approval, and constantly fear being blackballed."

THE INGREDIENTS FOR SUCCESS

In view of the recognized need for more and better qualified faculty in schools of nursing, one might reasonably expect that schools employing nurses new to academia would exert considerable effort to ensure that these neophytes undergo a socialization process designed to help them become successful in their new role. But, as the remark above demonstrates, this expectation is not always met. In fact, our thesis is that success in the role of nurse faculty member, when it does occur, is an unintended result of socialization.

Success in this role means building one's reputation as a teacher and a scholar; publishing original work; engaging in research; meriting favorable review by peers in one's department; being a skilled clinician; and in general meeting those criteria which have been established for achieving promotion and tenure. There are, of course, some who try on the academic role who are not suited to it because they have neither the intellectual ability nor the attitude toward learners that is essential for success. But in our view those neophytes who possess the potential for achieving success should be given the guidance and support necessary to enable them to fulfill that potential.

Socializing a person for any role essentially consists of transmitting to him the norms and values appropriate to actualizing the role. For nurses and others who are being socialized into academia, the process should also include identifying the criteria for promotion and attainment of tenure and helping them to progress toward meeting these criteria. Those guarding the portals can, if they wish, facilitate the neophyte's admission to their ranks as peers in a body of equals.

In reality, however, the socialization process is quite different from these ideal-typical assumptions. Among the variables affecting the process are: the nature of the organization; the congruence of members' and the organization's goals; and objective reality.

ORGANIZATIONAL CONSTRAINTS

The neophyte faculty member faces at least two major problems: she must define her own role and she must determine how that role fits into the organization. While a contract with the school or college may specify certain work expectations, and the courses one is assigned to teach may help to define others, these are far from complete guides to the entire scope of the faculty role.

The fact is that the organization (the university) is a system in itself and roles of members comprise a subsystem. Within that subsystem each faculty member is involved in a series of role transactions which are part of the energy exchange within the system in its goal-directedness.[2] One of the frustrations of the neophyte faculty within the university may well be created by their lack of understanding that the organization, as a system, has goals which are independent of those that are overtly defined in its bulletins and public pronouncements.

For example, a decision to offer two summer sessions rather than the usual one may be made at one level so as to generate income. This decision is then transmitted to each school or department and reflected in various ways. Faculty may be pressured to offer one or more courses; registrars may have to increase their staff; building services may be forced to alter schedules; security procedures will need to be revised or augmented; the food service which would have been closed down for several weeks may have to remain open; and so forth. While the decision may be rational in terms of the university's goals, it is not essential to the stated goal of offering high quality education.

This is but one example of many decisions initiated at various levels within the system that can result in the faculty member's having to expend added time and energy. If she had planned to engage in research during the summer—which she needs to do if she is to be promoted—she may find herself faced with strong peer pressure to teach an additional course and forgo her research. And if the pressure comes from a senior faculty member who will later participate in her review for promotion, she may find it irresistible.

GOAL CONGRUENCY

The second factor to be examined is the extent to which the organization's goals and the member's goals are congruent. There is no imperative that the goals of both parties are congruent in all respects; all that is necessary for a functioning system is that the employee within an organization recognize that the organization's goals are legitimate and that she make a moral contract not to impede movement toward those goals. To perform well in a role, it is more important that a person's expectations be congruent with those of others in the same role set than that she subscribe to the goals of the organization as a whole.[3] For example, if two faculty members are jointly responsible for a course, it is more important that their perceptions of their teaching goals be similar than that they agree with the university's fiscal policy.

The matter of values and the extent to which they are shared may be much more important than the matter of goals. This is especially true for organizations which employ professionals rather than unskilled or semiskilled workers. The professional is committed first to his profession and second to the employing organization. The nurse faculty member looks not only to her peers in the academic setting but also to those in the practice setting for role validation. No wonder, then, that nurse faculty are increasingly insisting on time to improve their clinical competence as a necessary adjunct to their role as teachers.

In many academic settings, however, this insistence may be a source of serious value conflict. If the all-university body which grants promotion or tenure does not equate clinical practice with scholarly achievement, the faculty member who devotes much of her time to this practice will find herself at a disadvantage when she is a candidate for promotion. While clinical practice indeed does not equate with such acknowledged scholarly activity as writing a book, it is nonetheless an essential component of an applied discipline such as nursing, medicine, or social work. No single individual has the resources to reconcile the values involved in this conflict; it is a problem calling for the joint efforts of nurse faculty and their colleagues from other disciplines. This value incongruency is undoubtedly one of the more important sources of role conflict for the neophyte who finds herself denied recognition for the expertise which was largely the basis for offering her a faculty position in the first place.

OBJECTIVE REALITY

The third factor to be considered is objective reality: that set of norms and values that the neophyte nurse faculty member discovers as she seeks to actualize her role. We use this term deliberately to distinguish between the real world-as-is and the ideal model-as-described before the individual takes on the faculty role.

In the ideal model all faculty are peers; each individual's opinion is valued as much as any other's; decisions are arrived at in a collegial fashion; rationality pervades discussion of controversial issues; each faculty member is allowed—even expected—to make her contribution to that particular area of curriculum in which she is interested or best prepared; each is expected to be a role model for students; each is encouraged to institute innovations in the teaching-learning process; and her performance is judged by her effectiveness as a teacher. In addition, although the contract letter may specify that faculty are expected to engage in research and contribute to the community, one's assigned course load and student contact hours are the salient demands of the new roles.

How does this ideal conception differ from objective reality? Although all faculty are peers, "senior" and "junior" are adjectives frequently used in conversations about faculty; these suggest a bi-level rather than unitary body. In the supposedly rational, collegial discussions which take place at department or course group levels, it becomes apparent that while the opinions of all faculty may be valued in so far as they are heard, the opinions of the senior faculty are valued somewhat more than those of the junior faculty. And, if one does not perceive the meaning of this initially, it is likely to become clear when one learns that on occasion outspoken junior faculty who are, in fact, good teachers have been passed over for promotion or tenure.

In regard to teaching, the neophyte faculty member discovers that the energy she has to expend to establish herself as a competent teacher leaves her exhausted, or nearly so. Moreover, rather than merely stepping from an office to a nearby classroom to which students obligingly come to listen (and, possibly, to learn), she must expend energy traveling to and from the sites where she has contact with students. Ultimately, or so one is led to believe, members of the senior faculty will assess the merits of her teaching. In reality, however, judgment of her contribution to knowledge and effectiveness as a teacher is rendered by the sole recipients of the teaching: the students. The basis for recognition from peers consists, in reality, of committee work, visibility, and occasionally verbosity. Research and contributions to the community assume the image of a menacing giant, since the time required even to consider how one might become engaged in research or what type of community activity one might select is unavailable.

How well the new faculty member understands all three variables—the nature of the organization, congruency of members' and organization goals, and objective reality—influences her success. Ideally, the socialization process should provide this understanding. Of the three variables, objective reality surfaces most frequently in daily activities where the socialization process occurs. At the outset of taking on the faculty role, objective reality takes priority for the individual over concern for the nature of the organization and the congruency of goals. After all, if a teacher cannot conduct a class for which she is solely responsible, understanding the nature of the organization will not be of much comfort or assistance to her.

DEALING WITH REALITY

Let us examine the process of socialization from the subjective perspective of the faculty member herself. The demands of objective reality are not explicit; in fact, it may take up to two years for the neophyte faculty member to recognize that they constrain her performance. True, expectations of her role may be discussed at the time of the employment interview. However, such hindrances as anxiety, not knowing the appropriate questions to ask, and maintaining her presence may all prevent her from remembering useful information.

The actual working environment adds multiple stimuli and increases exposure to objective reality. While the university's expectation of productivity in teaching, research and service is known to the neophyte, the teaching role is the one that commands her entire attention. Even so, it is not easy to implement that role fully during the faculty member's initial years. Her vision of the "ideal" role of university professor is likely to vanish when she finds herself struggling for survival with only one-third of that role actualized.

During the initial experiences as nurse educator, one's energy is consumed not so much by the teaching itself as by the mechanics of managing students, the public relations necessary at the clinical site, preparation of lectures, conducting discussions, and planning clinical assignments. Committee and ad hoc task force activities usurp what little physical and intellectual energy may remain.

A neophyte faculty member's previous socialization experience in graduate school or in the clinical service setting is very likely to have provided her with a value and reward system different from that prevailing in the academic setting. Graduate education in nursing, by and large, does not provide enough opportunities to acquire values and behaviors associated with the role of university professor.[4] Generally speaking, the institutional values that operate in the clinical service setting mean that staff are rewarded for conformity to routine rather than for innovation—also, that they acquire status and position by having authority delegated to them in the organizational hierarchy. The professional value system of the university, on the other hand, is such that faculty are rewarded for expertise in a given cognate subject area and status and position are acknowledged by the professional group rather than by some authority figure in the hierarchy.[5] Obviously, neither graduate school nor the clinical service setting prepares for the realities of the faculty role. There are, of course, some expectations commonly held for the professional in both the clinical setting and in the university—commitment to the service ideal, as well as to teaching and to publishing. Primary obligations differ, however. For the clinician it is the patient who commands her expert ability; for the faculty member, it is the student.

Ordinarily, during the first week of the academic year, considerable effort is invested in an orientation program for new faculty, part of which is directed to imparting the governing value system. This initial attempt to socialize neophyte faculty frequently results in information overload by the second week. As the faculty member sorts and sifts through the volumes of information she has heard, she tends to remember two general categories of facts necessary for day-to-day survival: the teaching assignment (What will I teach? Where will I teach?) and personal affairs (Who has the key to my office? How do I activate my health insurance? Where and when will a paycheck arrive?). All facts communicated in orientation regarding tenure, the research-teaching-service triad, the university, and the organization of the school are soon forgotten because they are not immediately useful to survival.

DISCOVERY-OVERLOAD SYNDROME

Attendance at faculty and departmental meetings, astute observations, and casual conversation—all these help socialize the neophyte faculty during the first few months and tend to increase her ability to participate intelligently in discussions and decision making. As junior faculty produce and participate, senior faculty come to accept them. Then the "disovery-overload" syndrome results. That is, as the faculty member's intelligence and ability are discovered by her colleagues, she becomes overloaded with invitations to serve on committees and task forces, with requests for consultation in clinical and crisis situations, and expected attendance at various functions. Until the neophyte becomes aware of this syndrome, her sense of relief at being accepted may land her with five committee appointments and 20 hours of consultation within one week!

Our speculation is that getting caught in the discovery-overload syndrome stems from political naiveté. Previous socialization and inexperience generate assumptions which are invalid in the new role. For example, a neophyte faculty member may assume that someone in an administrative role monitors her activities to prevent overload, not realizing that requests come independently from individuals who have no idea of the number of demands that others are making. Because previous socialization in the clinical service setting leads one to believe that a specific person is responsible for assigning tasks, the individual somewhat tardily realizes that in the academic setting one functions as an independent agent responsible for monitoring oneself.

The discovery-overload syndrome operates in a cyclic pattern. The faculty member sees her own interests and ideas reflected in the organization's activities and the faculty's decisions. This positive reinforcement increases self-confidence and retards breaking from the pattern. For example, when she has attended an out-out-town conference and responded to inquiries about her school's modus operandi, she feels important and worthwhile. What follows, though, is that as she becomes more active and productive, she gains further recognition from her peers, and then gets more involved, and the cycle continues, until suddenly she reaches the limit of her resources. Time, energy, and cognitive skills become totally committed to school activities, and her life revolves around the curriculum and related faculty activities. Hours spent in her office increase, and weekends may be entirely absorbed by preparation for next week's activities. Little, if any, time is available for recharging herself.

Bombardment by senior faculty with "you should do that" and "it will look good in your folder" runs concurrent with discovery-overload. This type of casual comment is meant to convey the requisites for success, but attempting to absorb all of the relevant information regarding tenure requirements together with facing the almost insurmountable task of producing in the research-teaching-service triad can be overwhelming. Any reasonable perspective on one's role within the organization gets lost in the flurry of daily activities demanded for survival. If, by chance, the faculty member does maintain a functional perspective on her role, the logistics of implementation may quickly consume the energy and time that should be available for productivity. How, for example, does one cope in a university where junior faculty must carry a 100 percent teaching workload during her first three years of employment? In the two years remaining for one to fulfill the additional tenure requirements, hopes for success are extinguished, since this is not enough time to produce anything substantive.

HOW NEW FACULTY COPE

At some point in the socialization process, the neophyte faculty member completely comprehends the expectations and demands of academia.

Among the possible responses are: a change in behavior, "burning out," and efforts to monitor and control the workload.

A change in behavior can limit exposure to requests impinging on one's time and energy. For example, a faculty member can decrease her visibility on campus by increasing her involvement in a setting removed from the school—the clinical setting. She can spend more hours than necessary there, read in the library, or claim attendance at off-campus functions. She can stop answering interoffice memos and keep her opinions to herself at meetings.

The second mode of reacting—making no attempt to negotiate role demands—results in fatigue, frustration, and disappointment. No time or energy remains for recovery; thus one attempts to sustain a high level of activity and "burns out." The person feels a lack of completeness with each task, a void of knowledge, and a yearning for personal development and enjoyment.

Neither of these responses moves neophyte faculty in the direction of success. A change in behavior allows the individual to rest as it decreases stimuli; however, it also limits opportunities for fulfilling the expectations for success. Becoming "burned out" consumes energy to the extent that even daily activities are an intolerable burden and the person is left drained. A possible consequence is that she seeks another environment and a different role.

The mode most conducive to success involves the faculty member's using her understanding of the situation to monitor and control the workload. She must be assertive enough to say "no" to others' requests, an action that surprises colleagues and may require repetition. To the extent that she knows her own abilities and interests and maintains a functional perspective on the role, she can select activities that are stimulating, satisfying, and appropriate to success. Coping is facilitated when one feels a sense of control over the situation, rather than feeling controlled by daily role demands. When such control is achieved, energy can then be directed to gaining an understanding of the organization and role and to planning a functional and feasible course of action.

Socialization, as currently conceived and as we have described it, almost assures the nonsuccess of the neophyte faculty member. Schlotfeldt has stated, "Nursing needs to seek out and develop its bright, probably rebellious, innovative young people and cultivate their leadership potentials."[6] Certainly the current mode of socialization does not acknowledge this imperative. If the bright, innovative, young nurses are to be cultivated for future leadership roles, then a better way must be found to accomplish this. A thoughtfully planned socialization process could assure more successes in the socialization of faculty and possibly decrease the number of comments such as the one quoted at the beginning of this article.

PLANNED SOCIALIZATION

Success in an academic career undoubtedly is a goal for most neophyte faculty members and for the organizations employing them. Not all of those employed will remain, however. Some may decide that teaching is not the career for them; others may not be able to fulfill the criteria for achieving promotion and tenure. What can be done to retain and support those professionals who have both the ability and the desire to become scholars? A planned socialization process could help prevent the loss of potentially able scholars.

Planned socialization, in our view, at least, should address at least three important issues: the need for information, the political naiveté of neophytes, and the assignment or selection of mentors. The first of these—information giving—becomes more effective if information is provided in the order in which the new faculty need it. Information about tenure requirements, organizational structure, and expectations about research, although necessary for success, constitutes noncritical material for the neophyte faculty member during her first six months of employment. She needs first of all to learn how to deal with her teaching assignment, how to cope with ordinary demands of students, and how to become acquainted with the clinical setting. Short, informal sessions dealing with other important information, accompanied by written materials, should be arranged for the second semester of employment. Such meetings could serve the dual function of allowing some discussion among faculty about the problems encountered during their first semester's experience.

The neophyte faculty member is politically naive in dealing with her role and the organization. Besides not knowing where power and influence reside, she may also lack familiarity with the system and the extent to which it allows freedom or imposes limitations on her role. Open, honest discussions on how to deal with the system plus some opportunity to meet persons who are influential can expedite the development of political awareness.

In addition, the neophyte needs assistance in finding a mentor within the senior faculty. According to Sheehy, finding a mentor is an important developmental task during an early stage of adult life.[7] That is, success in a professional role can be facilitated by a relationship with someone familiar with the role who can answer questions, discuss issues, and give feedback. It seems that most opportunities for discussion occur during small group situations such as course meetings where junior faculty associate only with other junior faculty. Some problem situations for junior faculty could be averted if a more experienced person were readily available for consultation at such times.

Establishing a relationship with a mentor is basically establishing an exchange based on trust. The junior faculty member who is initially ill at ease in the presence of a highly qualified, knowledgeable person learns new role responses, while the senior attempts to cope with the threatening feelings of being replaced or pushed out of her position by someone younger—and perhaps intellectually superior.

Once the relationship is established, the mentor can help in planning the workload, providing social encounters with other senior faculty, sharing teaching materials, and providing information on the politics of the school or department. A mentor relationship offers benefits to both parties; the gratitude of the junior for the help received and the senior's gratification in having her expertise and wisdom recognized pave the way for a continuing social exchange. If common interests exist, joint research projects may be a further fruitful outcome. In addition, the concerns and questions of the junior faculty members may stimulate interest and learning in the senior faculty member. The benefits received and enjoyed by both parties are likely to lead to the development of a strong collegial relationship extending to other members of the faculty.

To the extent that the circumstances we have chronicled represent accurately the characteristic way in which nurse faculty are socialized, the process leaves much to be desired. Failure to transmit clearly the norms of a particular social environment not only puts the new teacher at a disadvantage in her attempt to take on the appropriate role, but may even doom her to failure. One must practice a role in order to be successful at it. Prerequisite to such practice is an accurate conception of those behavioral expectations and demands which constitute the role and which are shared by members of the role set.

Recognition of the fact that the prevailing mode of socialization within academic nursing is less than optimal may stimulate re-examination of that process. Following that, the process can be altered so that it is more directly related to the desired outcome—that is, successful socialization. Explicit attempts to bring about a degree of value consensus would seem to be essential for those faculties where such a consensus does not now exist.

To some extent the value issue is one of the aspects of academia that affects nursing (and other applied disciplines) in a special way, since, unlike the humanities, nursing must establish its credibility in two domains rather than one: the practice arena and the academy. If faculty are divided in the value they attach to one or the other of these domains, a potential problem exists in terms of the quality of teaching and the quality of scholarship among the faculty themselves.

Nursing's legitimacy as a profession depends upon its ability to demonstrate superior competence in both of these domains, and it cannot do so unless it pays greater attention to the socialization of new teachers. If the faculty of a given school wish to see that school ranked among the acknowledged best in the university, the socialization of each new faculty member must become a concern of the corporate body.

REFERENCES

1. Nursing Outlook. NEWS AND REPORTS: Nurse Faculty Census Shows Higher Employment. 25:296, May 1977.
2. Conway, M.E.: Organizations, professional autonomy, and role relationships. In Hardy, M. and Conway, M. (eds.): *Role Theory: Perspectives for the Health Professionals.* New York, Appleton-Century-Crofts, 1978.
3. Merton, R.: *Social Theory and Social Structure.* New York, Free Press, 1968, p.44.
4. Batey, M.V.: The two normative worlds of the university nursing faculty. *Nursing Forum,* 8:13, 1969.
5. Williamson, J.A.: The conflict-producing role of the professionally socialized nurse-faculty member. *Nursing Forum,* 11:358-359, 1972.
6. Schlotfeldt, R.M.: Educator. An oral history interview. In Safier, G. (ed.): *Contemporary American Leaders in Nursing: An Oral History.* New York, McGraw-Hill Book Co., 1977, p. 347.
7. Sheehy, Gail: *Passages: Predictable Crises of Adult Life.* New York, E.P. Dutton and Co., 1976, pp. 27, 131.

7

Developing Staff Research Potential

Overcoming Nurse Resistance to Research

Joanne S. Stevenson

In some fields of study it is safe to assume that a learner is positively disposed toward becoming a researcher. In nursing, however, the contrary is more often true: nurses do not visualize themselves as potential researchers. Because the pervading concept of a nurse is almost an antithesis to the traditional image of a researcher, nursing activities and research activities are viewed as alien to each other. Research is a hard, objective, and unfeeling enterprise; nursing is a nurturing, intuitive, physically and emotionally supportive enterprise. How can one person engage in both practices without becoming a traitor to one of them? Even more mystifying is the dilemma of how to apply an objective measurement approach to the subjective world of nursing without destroying the phenomena that are being studied. Finally, there is the secret belief that nurse-researchers are a special breed.

The most difficult hurdle faced by teachers, administrators, and staff developers committed to enhancing the research capability of professional nurses is changing nurses' self-images and occupational images to include research. One clinical specialist expressed her personal struggle this way: "How do you get the urge? Do you get a special calling or what? Will it ruin me as a clinical specialist?" Translated into the jargon of a planned change model, the question should be: "How does one become free from the restraining forces and immersed in the change forces?"

This article will deal with the following interrelated topics: (1) a basic philosophy about development of nurses and nursing students who evidence aptitude for research; (2) introduction of Lewin's framework for planned change to guide the metamorphosis of nurses from self-discounting research-resisters to committed, practicing investigators; (3) presentation of selected strategies and tactics to progress from stage to stage in the change

73

process; (4) presentation of peer group strategy to effect major attitude adjustment; (5) a description of peer group activities from beginning to end of the research proposal development process; (6) maintenance of the peer group through all the stages of project implementation, analysis, and reporting; and (7) ripple effects to other staff. The first four topics are dealt with in this chapter; the last three will be discussed in Chapter 8.

POSITION ON RESEARCH DEVELOPMENT

The author's basic philosophy about development of research potential among nurses can be summarized in two simple ideas—early identification and "tough love."

Students who show promise in those cognitive and psychomotor dimensions usually associated with successful research performance ought to be identified early in their undergraduate program and introduced to nurse-researchers. Research assistantships, group and independent studies, as well as formal research courses, are useful mechanisms for involving undergraduate and early graduate students in a research project that does not overwhelm or discourage them. Promising staff nurses, head nurses, and clinical specialists can be exposed to a parallel approach. Service agencies may not be able to add a full-time nurse-researcher to their staff, but many could afford the services of a long-term research consultant to function as the research mentor and group facilitator with the agency nursing staff. The consultant could help the group plan and implement one or more studies of its choosing.

Criteria for identifying research aptitude have long been available, but nursing administrators and educators are just realizing their responsibility to use them. Much of the prediction activity that has taken place to date has focused on the clinical specialty choice, the leadership potential, or the managerial and educational potential of the target group. Only in rare instances were nurses who showed high research aptitude so informed.

Nursing schools accept applicants with superior scholastic records and regularly graduate scores of nurses with superior academic records. Yet, the majority of these graduates go off to jobs in nursing where their superior intelligence is viewed as undesirable by physicians or the bureaucratic hierarchy. As in other fields comprised primarily of women, many of them survive in the system by unwittingly discounting their intelligence. They stop reading professional literature and develop apathetic attitudes about new trends in nursing. Hidden among the nursing staffs of the health care organizations in this country are countless nurses who have far more intellectual talent than they need to fulfill current functions. Many of them would break out of their protective shell of apathy if they could become involved in something stimulating and inherently fulfilling. Clinical nursing research is an activity which meets this requirement very well.

The second basic component of this philosophy is "tough love." It is an expression used in lay self-help groups to denote the use of leveling and confrontation. When people are resisting personal growth, resisting their responsibility to mature, and resisting personal change, it is dysfunctional for others to reinforce or legitimize this resistance. While sympathy and empathy from others provide immediate comfort, they justify the person's remaining in the non-growth state. The more useful behavior is to refuse to participate in maintaining the status quo. Leveling and confrontation may cause hurt feelings momentarily, but these tactics tend to jolt the person into self-realization which later can lead to growth. Nurses are notorious for nursing co-workers—for example, physicians, hospital administrators, and other nurses. Nursing of other nurses often is manifested as reinforcing their stagnation behavior by agreeing with their excuses for resisting change. "Tough love" is predicated on the belief that it is the responsibility of educators, administrators, and staff-developers to promote growth in staff members, rather than to ignore and thus excuse and reinforce stagnation. Honesty does not come easily to women nurses because they have been socialized to be deferent, tactful, and indirect communicators.[1] It is difficult for a nurse to tell another nurse (subordinate, peer, or even nursing student) that she has a special talent such as research aptitude that is being wasted. Were administrators to take a hard look at their agency staff members, they would discover a surprising number of superior intellects left to atrophy.

PLANNED CHANGE

So what can administrators and staff developers do to rehabilitate and to facilitate growth in these dormant intellects? Lewin's framework for planned change is easy to learn and to use.[2] The framework lends itself well to the generation of a variety of strategies and tactics; when a change agent tries something that fails an alternative is easy to generate. Lewin proposed that the process of planned change be conceptualized as consisting of three sequential stages or states in the target system (which in this case consists of one or more nurses with dormant research aptitude): unfreezing, changing, and refreezing. These three system states are observable and thus serve to measure progress or to signal a need for recycling.

Unfreezing

The first stage is the most difficult to initiate. To unfreeze a target system, the force of inertia (status quo) must be overcome and the potential energies stored in the target system must be transformed into active energy for change. A stable system is not apt to embrace the tumult brought on by a major change. A system that is already in crisis, or frustrated with the status quo, is more likely to embrace the prospect of change. Unfreezing a complacent system frequently means stimulating it to the end of producing a crisis or arousing dissatisfaction with the status quo or both.

The unfreezing strategies most often used in bureaucratic organizations are the power-coercive mode and the legal-bureaucratic mode.[3] Either of these modes is likely to produce a crisis vis-a-vis anxiety about status in the organization. The power-coercive mode can be expressed as subtle or overt threats about loss, such as loss of position or loss of power and prestige. It can also be expressed by withholding rewards, such as merit raises, promotions or special privileges. The legal-bureaucratic mode might consist of referring to external requirements that stipulate certain changes must take place. One example would be stating that the Joint Commission on Hospital Accreditation requires the change. Either of these modes can successfully produce unfreezing, but, unfortunately, they can also produce fear and resentment that may take a long time to resolve.

The strategy most widely used in more egalitarian groups is the normative-re-educative mode.[4] Consciousness raising, one tactic in the normative-re-educative mode, is frequently used as the first step in the unfreezing process. An excellent initial tactic, it can continue to be useful throughout the change process. Consciousness raising can be haphazard and opportunistic, or it can be a well-devised multi-faceted plan to bombard the target system with several rounds of relevant information and periodic reinforcements about the negative aspects of the status quo.[5] This tactic works best if other people or events in the environment are also emitting congruent signals. A multi-stimulus approach creates a cycle, beginning with a heightened awareness that promotes more acute observation. This leads to the intake of further knowledge from the environment concerning the subject, which leads in turn to more acute attention when the next round of consciousness raising occurs. The cycle continues until there is evidence that unfreezing is well along, and that at least some people are willing to begin the change process. In this instance, unfreezing means that an aggregate of nurses become aware of their dormant talents. The goal for the change stage will eventually be defined by each nurse. However, since this article is about the development of hidden research potential, that will be the stated goal for the change process.

Changing

As noted earlier, nurses find it extremely difficult to define themselves as potential researchers. One-to-one tutoring usually fails to produce the desired redefinition of self. Peer groups work better because they are effective, efficient, and fun. They are efficient in that one research mentor can work with 8 to 14 partially unfrozen nurses in each group. Peer groups are effective; that is, they do produce measurable change in their members. However, not every group organized to become a peer group will actually develop into one.

The forces moving toward change in the peer group include: group dynamics; alteration of role relationships; shared examination of childhood stereotypes about women, nurses, and nursing; and the reinforcement resulting from small successes among the budding investigators. In the first group session, individuals often recognize their own devaluing attitudes about women and nurses in the expressions of others. Members help each other ferret out false assumptions about themselves that they have absorbed from significant others. One group member may express a complete lack of confidence in her ability to participate in a research study and may be confronted by a peer about discounting herself. Another peer may say the person has excellent aptitude for research and may present data to back up the judgment. Such leveling and confrontation are encouraged because they promote an honest, open communication style that is necessary here for growth and later for the development of true collaborative relationships in the research enterprise.

The facilitator's task throughout the life of the group is to serve as role model, discussion leader, and research mentor. In the first few sessions, the facilitator's major task is to heighten awareness of out-dated or erroneous beliefs about the self, women, nurses, nursing, and the scientific method. New information is supplied by the facilitator as group members replace old beliefs with tentative new conceptions.

The peer group serves as a relatively safe test area for heavily socialized nurses to discover the inaccuracy of what they were taught to believe, to work through the period of resentment and hostility, to accept the past as part of the evolution of women and of nurses, and to begin constructive use of their new-found potential.

In most instances where the facilitator believes in "tough love," the peer group will spend no more than four to six sessions on the foregoing processes. A group that spends too much time bemoaning the past may stop growing. One useful approach is to spend part of every group session on some content related to the research process. Eventually, the primary emphasis shifts from examining and reframing attitudes to developing basic research knowledge and skills.

Peer group work on the research enterprise itself can take several different approaches. For instance, the group must decide whether it will work together on one project or members will work on separate projects according to their personal interests. Such decisions should be made rationally but expeditiously, so that the more substantive phases of research development can proceed.

SUMMARY

Chapter 7 dealt with overcoming the most difficult and time-consuming part of research development work in nursing, the heavy resistance of nurses to research development attempts on their behalf. A basic philosophy about research development was presented, followed by Lewin's model of planned change, which is comprised of three stages: unfreezing, changing, and refreezing. Three strategies for unfreezing were presented and discussed briefly. Assuming that unfreezing was successful, the discussion moved to strategies for the change process. The peer group approach was chosen as a prototypic strategy because it has a better success rate than other approaches and is the most suitable strategy for the majority of situations involving nonstudents. In situations where feasible, research apprenticeships may be more successful than peer groups. It was suggested that a few early meetings of the peer group be devoted to an analysis of basic assumptions, values, and beliefs about women, nursing, and research. Concurrently, the peer group was to be started on a concrete agenda directed toward learning and implementing the research process.

Chapter 8 will describe the functioning of the peer group during each phase of the research planning process and the research implementation process. Finally, refreezing in the change state will be discussed in terms of signals of readiness in the target system, strategies for refreezing, termination of the peer group, and other relevant issues.

REFERENCES

1. Lakoff, R.: *Language and Woman's Place*. New York, Harper Colophon Books, 1975.
2. Lewin, K.: *Field Theory in Social Studies*. New York, Harper and Row, 1951, pp. 188–237.
3. Smoyak, S.A.: Toward understanding nursing situations: A transaction paradigm. *Nursing Research*, 18:405–411, 1969.
4. Chin, R. and Benne, K. D.: General strategies for effecting changes in human systems. In Bennis, W. G., Benne, K. D. and Chin, R. (eds.): *The Planning of Change*. 3rd ed. New York, Holt, Rinehart, and Winston, 1961, pp. 22–45.
5. Alinsky, S. D.: *Rules for Radicals*. New York, Vintage Books, 1972.

8

Developing Staff Research Potential

Planning & Implementing Studies

Joanne S. Stevenson

In Chapter 7, four of seven points relating to the development of staff research potential were discussed. These four points were: (1) a basic philosophy about development of nurses who evidence aptitude for research; (2) a framework for staff research development—we used Lewin's framework of planned change, which defines three stages: unfreezing, changing, and refreezing[1]; (3) strategies to guide nurses toward positive attitudes about themselves as developing researchers; and (4) a rationale for choosing the small peer group as a means of developing research proposals among neophyte nurse-investigators.[2]

This chapter presents three additional points relevant to developing staff research potential: utilization of the peer group approach through all stages of the research process; description of peer group activities from problem identification through proposal writing and on into project implementation; and the refreezing process, wherein these nurses develop long-term commitments to research as part of their career goals. These seven points are equally relevant whether the nursing staff are members of service agencies or are faculty members in academic settings.

Chapter 7 discussed the use of peer group meetings for unfreezing nurses from long-standing attitudes of negativity toward research or inadequate feelings about themselves as researchers. In these sessions, they struggle to redefine themselves as nurse-practitioners or nurse-educators who could also become nurse-investigators. In addition to this resocializing process, the peer group meetings include content-focused experiences that begin with problem identification and go through the planning and development of the research proposal. In this article, we describe this content-focused portion of the peer group meetings. In Chapter 7 the functions of the group facilitator were described as those of research mentor, discussion leader, group processor, and research role model.[3] The facilitator should be a trained, experienced researcher with some background in small group methods.[4]

LEARNING THROUGH DOING

Development of research competence within a peer group can best begin after time as been spent discussing members' attitudes toward themselves as potential nurse-investigators and about nursing's unmet responsibility to add to the body of scientific knowledge. The specific tactics used to introduce research content, as well as the nature and level of that content, depends on the composition of the group. Different tactics will be required for *educationally homogeneous groups than for heterogeneous groups.* Educationally mixed groups probably are handled better when highly educated members are teamed with partners having less education. Consider two prototypic groups: one is composed of persons with divergent research interests and varying amounts of research training. Another is composed primarily of persons with little research training or experience. The members of either group may choose to develop individual research projects, two- to three-person team projects, or to work as a group on one project with a qualified group member or the facilitator serving as principal investigator. In this article, the discussion will be limited to individual research projects or team projects involving two or three group members. Projects involving the entire group are described in the literature.[5,6]

The basic approach to group work presented here is *learning through doing.* There is minimal lecturing. Most lecturing is extemporaneous—in response to the situation. Textbook materials are used by members only when needed. Members are advised to read several sources on one topic when they need the information to make decisions about any step in the proposal development process. The discussion content in group sessions focuses on the research projects under development by group members: textbook material is background information only.

Research Proposal as Both
Process and Product

Since this article focuses on the development of nurse-investigators under the aegis of intra-agency* development, the strategies used throughout are

---

*Intra-agency development could mean staff development, continuing education, or it could refer to the efforts made by schools, agencies, or regional organizations funded by external sponsors or by internal resources to upgrade the research capabilities of their nursing faculty or nursing staff.

based on a normative-reeducative mode. [7,8] Successful application of this mode requires that members become involved in the social system of the group so that they become committed to the group's goals and continue to participate in the group's evolution even during high stress periods, in the face of negative sanctions from significant persons outside the group, or during frustrating periods in the development of their project. Although the specifics may differ, every group will experience such stresses. In general, the facilitator can expect members to have individual difficulties to overcome, and sometimes the group itself hits a high stress period. Riding out these difficulties is part of the socialization process. Success will strengthen the group members' resolve to continue the research development process.

In the method advocated here, the facilitator conveys to the group the expectation that members will act as consultants and peer reviewers for each other in discussions about each other's research projects and that they will support each other when problems arise in the proposal development process. The group is thus readied to move ahead with development of specific research projects.

The content portion of a group session might go as follows: Several wide blackboards or a tablet of blank newsprint is shared among members. Each person or team describes in one sentence the problem to be studied and presents it to the group. Group members and the facilitator ask clarifying questions, suggest ways the problem statement can be written up, suggest conceptual bases or theoretical frameworks that seem to fit the problem and the verbalized goals, and make suggestions about further work to be done before the next group meeting. *Every research project should get a brief hearing at this session.*

The approach can vary at subsequent sessions. One approach is to have most or all studies presented and discussed briefly during each session. Following this approach, the primary focus of the next sessions is on subsequent steps of the research planning process; for example, one session may focus on developing theoretical frameworks for the research projects, another on constructing the objectives or hypotheses, still another on writing operational definitions of the major variables and finding ways of measuring them. Each research project is discussed in relation to the step of the research process agreed upon for that day. This approach helps keep group members parallel in development and up-to-date on peers' work.

Another approach is to have one or two research projects discussed in depth at each session, so that each one is presented as an integrated whole. (This approach works well for sophisticated researchers who need only one or a few sessions with peers for review or consultation. It has distinct disadvantages when used with a group of neophytes who are developing research knowledge and skills at the same time they are developing a research project.)

Proposal development is periodically difficult and frustrating. Problems often arise during work on the theoretical framework, operational definitions, measurement of variables, and data analysis plan. Members should have access to the facilitator, another consultant, or more experienced fellow members between sessions. Particularly noteworthy are the beneficial effects seen when group members take formal research courses concurrent with the group development efforts. Courses about specific research methods or analytic techniques add vitality and depth to the total group effort. Even one or two persons so involved will noticeably enhance the quality of peer suggestions made during the group sessions and between sessions.

Over the course of several weeks or months, the proposals continue to be developed and refined. Members assume responsibility for reading and developing drafts of parts of the proposals between sessions. During group meetings, all members share responsibility for activities related to each proposal: questioning, suggesting, critiquing, reinforcing, correcting, broadening, narrowing, encouraging, and praising. The session is exciting when several members actively discuss each research project; it is dull and frustrating when only the facilitator and the presenters hold two-way conversations about each project while the others sit in silence.

Sometimes a group will become overly zealous and provide too much advice or conflicting suggestions. Such behavior can confuse a particularly suggestible investigator. The group facilitator may have to caution the group from time to time about making unrealistic suggestions. Members thus become progressively more skilled at helping peers, rather than overburdening them with unrealistic suggestions.

Attention to Internal Consistency

A particularly useful tactic for preventing "proposal drift" is to use some form of internal consistency guide. "Proposal drift" refers to changes and inconsistencies that develop as parts of the research project come together. In a severe case of drift, parts of the project, such as the problem statement, the hypotheses, and the methods, are appropriate to three different studies rather than to one. Drift results from the influence of literature reviews that shift and reshift the investigator's thinking, from suggestions of various people, or simply from lack of attention to the logical progression of the research proposal.

An Internal Consistency Guide is shown in Figure 8.1. The facilitator would distribute such guides and each member would fill in the blank spaces with pertinent information about her research project. The guide helps an

Figure 8.1   Internal Consistency Guide

Problem Statement	Theoretical Framework	Method(s)	Data Analysis Plan	Outline of Findings	Targets for Recommen- dations
In *one* sentence, state the problem to be studied.	Outline the theory or theories that will be used to underpin study or list the assumptions.	If experimental— specify the design; if non-experimental— specify kind. Also, list major variables, instruments, or other data collection techniques.	What will collected data look like? Will analysis be statistical or not? Will it be non-parametric or parametric? What specific tests will be used?	Will findings be at level of trends because small convenience sample used? Will findings be directly applicable to care; are they at a basic level; or are they exploratory in nature?	Theory/ Research Possible implications for future research and theory testing or modification.
Objectives	Previous Research	Sampling Design			Practice
Describe broad objectives, specific aims, or even the hypotheses: 1. 2. 3. etc.	Outline types of research or specific studies that lead to this study; or outline the literature to be reviewed.	Describe whether sampling is random or convenience; report other sampling design specifications, such as how many groups, numbers in each group, methods of selection and assignment.			Action research and demonstration projects have direct practice implications. State possible recommendations.

investigator keep in touch with the major components of her project study at all times. It provides a brief overview that is easily altered, since everything is contained on one sheet of paper. Further, this guide provides a simple means of summarizing an entire research project on a classroom-size blackboard, making it available to the peer group involved in discussion. Later in the proposal development process, members can pass out filled-in copies for critique and discussion by the facilitator and group members.

As shown in Figure 8.1, headings in the guide correspond to sections of a typical research proposal. Other headings can be substituted or some can be eliminated. The purpose of the guide is to help achieve logical progression and congruence. Such a description of all the parts of a research study on a single sheet of paper helps both investigator and reviewer spot incongruities as they look across the columns. The investigator cannot depend solely on this device; working and reworking of the narrative proposal must proceed as well, but the guide serves as a synthesis of the major internal parts of a research proposal.

STEPS OF THE RESEARCH PROPOSAL

The steps involved in developing a complete research plan include the following (see Figure 8.1): (1) designation of the *problem* to be studied; (2) translation of the problem into *objectives*, research questions, or hypotheses; (3) designation of an acceptable *theoretical framework* that explains the investigator's orientation toward the research problem; (4) selection of a research method, whether experimental or nonexperimental; (5) specification of the research design, including sampling, instrumentation, treatment (if appropriate), and data collection techniques; (6) plans for the grouping and *analysis* of collected data; (7) visualization of how the findings might look; (8) decision on whether recommendations could be made about practice or about the next step in researching the problem; and finally (9) plans for dissemination of results to appropriate audiences. Not included in this list are: the rationale, the significance of the study, personnel qualifications and duties, and the budget. Consideration of these runs parallel to steps 2 through 6 and can be brought up for discussion by the facilitator when the members are ready for these pragmatic considerations.

The Problem Statement

Deciding on a problem to be studied is the logical first step for any would-be investigator. Problem identification can be achieved in several ways: a group member may bring a researchable question from the work situation; the group facilitator may stimulate discussion about researchable problems by handing out lists of priority areas prepared by recognized experts[9,10,11]; or group members can identify problems as they discuss their areas of nursing expertise or their major concerns about nursing practice, education, or administration. A few persons know precisely what they wish to study, but most begin with a vague topic area of problematic experience and must be helped to achieve greater specificity. The facilitator can encourage each member to become more specific with requests such as: "State the problem that you wish to study in one sentence. Name the specific thing you want *most* to study about this problem. List three hunches you have about how———(the named phenomenon) happens as it does." Members are encouraged to rethink their statements and refine them for the next group meeting. Group members quickly catch onto this tactic of helping themselves and their peers clarify, specify, and crystallize thinking. Such specifying tactics are then used in group sessions for each subsequent step of the research planning process.

During each meeting, topic-relevant readings are assigned. These are discussed at subsequent meetings, used by each member for proposal development, and used by the group for consultation to peers' projects.

Remaining Parts of the Proposal

The remaining steps of the proposal development process, while not simple, are relatively straightforward. Research textbooks adequately treat sampling and other design considerations. Further, consultants who can give advice on design and analysis are not difficult to locate. The wise facilitator will steer neophyte investigators away from complex research projects that require the creation of new methods or new analytic models. It is better for new investigators to develop projects that are manageable at their level of expertise and that make use of available designs and analytic procedures.

The same is true for data collection procedures. It is important that investigators develop habits of rigorous specification of the core elements of the plan—namely, the sampling procedures, the major variables, the instruments to be used to measure the variables, and the procedures for instrumentation. In experimental studies, one must clearly operationalize the experimental treatment (the new procedure or program to be tested) so that it will be applied consistently to all subjects and can be described in the final report for others to replicate. Whether planning an experimental or descriptive study, new investigators usually experience a greater sense of success if they use available instruments or experimental treatments that can be described in behavioral terms. The facilitator can be frank in explaining the above recommendations to group members and may even make ground rules to enforce them. Narrowing the parameters in this way is easily justified, both in terms of seeking positive research experiences for the investigators and building upon past research toward an integrated body of nursing science. Trail-blazing research efforts are better left to experienced researchers with a solid foundation in traditional methods of research and analysis.

Group members are encouraged to draft and redraft their written proposals. It is useful for the facilitator to read and critique partial drafts of the proposals between group meetings. The written drafts can also be circulated among group members, with each one responsible for giving feedback to the author(s).

Formal pilot studies may or may not be necessary. If the investigators are building on prior research, the need for instrument validations and other typical pilot activity should be minimal. At the same time, each study should have practice runs of the major procedures: sampling, informed consent, treatments, and data collection. Practice runs will bring to light vagaries, inadequacies, and impracticalities in the plan that can be resolved before the project gets under way.

FUNDING

Once proposal development work gets firmly under way, the search for potential funding sources becomes a priority. The facilitator or someone else knowledgeable about funding sources in the public and private sectors investigates possible funding sources for each of the developing studies. Internal funds of the agency or school, sources in the immediate locale, or foundations that give small grants are probably the best potential sponsors for first-time researchers.[12] However, the nature of a research project may require that it be sponsored for three or more years with a large annual budget. Usually, such a research project would be submitted to a federal agency or a national foundation.[13] In either case, contacts should be made with appropriate staff persons in the potential sponsor agencies well in advance of proposal submissions so that agency interest can be determined, questions answered, and proposals redrafted to include staff feedback.

IMPLEMENTATION

Waiting while submitted grants are in the review process can be tedious. Group members can be encouraged to take formal courses in research or statistics during this time. Group sessions will be held less frequently but not abandoned. Continued meetings are useful to maintain group cohesion, to keep interest sparked and, in particular, to further the resocialization process of changing nonresearchers into persons who are identified and who identify themselves as nurse-investigators. At least one session should be devoted to generating alternatives for each research project in case it should be disapproved. Group members may be actively involved in pilot testing one or more of their procedures. If so, some group sessions can be used for suggesting changes in problematic parts of the designs.

As decisions of the potential sponsors are received, the approved grantees become involved in a bevy of activity to get their research projects started.

Disapproved projects must be redesigned or submitted to other potential sponsors. Again, the continuing group meetings help keep both successful and unsuccessful grant applicants from losing confidence in themselves or in their project.

While they are implementing their research projects, the funded group should meet from time to time for progress reports, exchange of experiences, and advice. As each investigator or team approaches the end of their research project, they should present their entire study—including findings, conclusions, and recommendations—to peers for discussion and critique. This tactic provides practice and removes some of the anxiety associated with presenting one's first research paper before an audience of strangers. At least one session should focus on postresearch plans. What step logically follows the one being completed? How will the investigator complete a final written report of the current project? To which journals will manuscripts be submitted? Will a proposal be developed for a subsequent study? Have career plans changed or become crystallized? Is further education the next logical goal?

REFREEZING

Ideally, most of the nurses resocialized in the manner described in this article would be committed to research as an integral component of their career. Such a resocialization, called "refreezing," would constitute the third phase of the change process described in Lewin's framework.[14] Unfreezing was the melting of each person's original neutral or negative opinion about self as a potential investigator; changing was the process of learning to think and act like an investigator; refreezing means solidifying a new self-image that includes thinking and acting like an investigator from now on.

In reality, not all members will be resocialized. A few members will complete a single small study in order to fulfill some one-time motivation, and then they will forget about research. For this group, the first change phase—unfreezing—failed. Some members will decide to pursue formal education to improve their knowledge base and repertoire of research and analysis skills. Such persons became firmly tied to the change as they fulfill these goals, and they are likely to become "refrozen" in the self-image of nurse-researcher at some future time. The employer, whether a school or service agency, may temporarily (or permanently) lose such persons while they are pursuing educational goals. Agencies should understand that a short-term personnel cost accompanies successful research development programming.

There may be a third group composed of persons who are somewhere between the two extremes. They are positively disposed towards future research but are not committed enough to do anything more now. This group is still unfrozen and might benefit from a short rest. In time they can be invited into a new research development group where they can go through a second research experience. Such "second round" members add depth to a' group, since their previous experience can be used in the group process. If peer groups cease to exist and these still unfrozen persons are left alone, they may regress. A mailing or routing list can be used to circulate materials just often enough to give them a sense of staying in the informed circle while they are deciding whether to get involved in further research activities.

SYSTEM CHANGES IN THE AGENCY

An agency that commits time, money, and personnel to research development may want documentation that the total agency (school of nursing or nursing component of the service agency) benefited from the effort. Sometimes, beneficial effects are difficult to document except in terms of individual personnel upgrading. In an agency where four or five research projects are being implemented and four or five sets of faculty or staff are intimately involved, the effects may be noticeable throughout the system. There may be directly measurable effects on teaching or patient care. There will also be monetary effects from funded studies and publicity from presented papers and published articles. Finally, internal system effects manifest themselves through requests for the formation of new research development groups, for research workshops or other short-term approaches, and for research report conferences.

Research development is not a one-shot or short-term activity. It is a long-term process that begins with the use of unfreezing, change, and refreezing techniques on nurse faculty or staff. A peer group is the suggested medium through which these nursing personnel learn research project development. It is also the medium through which they start becoming resocialized to view themselves as nurse-investigators as well as nurse-practitioners, nurse-educators, or nurse-administrators.

REFERENCES

1. Lewin, K.: *Field Theory in Social Sciences*. New York, Harper and Row, 1951, pp. 188–237.
2. Stevenson, J. S.: Developing research potential of nursing staff. *Journal of Nursing Administration*, 8:44–46, 1978.

3. Stevenson, J. S.: 1978, pp. 45-46.
4. Lippitt, G.: *Visualizing Changes*. Fairfax, Va., NLT Learning Resources, 1973.
5. Lindemann, C. A. and Van Aernam, B. A.: Research program for nurses. *Hospitals,* 44: 89-91, 1970.
6. Lindemann, C. A.: Nursing research: a visible, viable component of nursing practice. *Journal of Nursing Administration,* 3:18-21, 1973.
7. Intra-agency development could mean staff development, continuing education, or it could refer to the efforts made by schools, agencies, or regional organizations funded by external sponsors or by internal resources to upgrade the research capabilities of their nursing faculty or nursing staff.
8. Chin, R. and Benne, K. D.: Gemera; strategies for effecting changes in human systems. In Bennis, W. C., Benne, K. D. and Chin, R. (eds.): *The Planning of Change.* 3rd ed. Chicago, Holt, Rinehart and Winston, 1976, pp. 22-45.
9. Abdellah, F. G.: U.S. Public Health Services contribution to nursing research—past, present, future. *Nursing Research,* 26:244-249, 1977.
10. Gortner, S. R., Bloch, D., and Phillips, T. P.: Contributions of nursing research to patient care. *Journal of Nursing Administration,* 6:22-28, 1976.
11. WICHE. Delphi Survey of Clinical Research Priorities. Final Report. Boulder, Co., WICHE, 1974.
12. Noe, L. (ed.): *The Foundation Grants Index, 1975.* New York, Columbia University Press, 1976.
13. Campos, R. G.: Securing information on funding sources for nursing research. *Journal of Nursing Administration,* 6:16-18, 54, 1976.
14. Lewin, K.: 1951.

III
Education for a Practitioner/ Teacher Role

Introduction

Lorraine Machan

The fact that some effective practitioner/teachers exist without having had the benefit of an education directing them toward this role as it is interpreted in Part I of this book may appear to some to negate the need for a curriculum model for educating practitioner/teachers. However, the most direct method to produce the large number of practitioner/teachers needed is to inspire the graduate student through the graduate program itself with the concept that views practice, teaching, and research as one multifaceted role. To do this the curriculum should assist the student to see the potential as well as the feasibility of the role, and should assist the student in developing role behaviors as well as providing basic knowledge essential for practice of the role.

Although the focus of this book is on the practitioner/teacher, the curriculum model provides a framework for role development, in general. For example, our curriculum also prepares practitioner/managers. By creating awareness in students of the unlimited possibilities that lie within the range of recombining role components and behaviors in new forms, a role-oriented program should provide a foundation for more effective emergence of new roles to meet the present and future needs of society.

The chapters in this unit are devoted to a description of both process and content utilized in educating graduate students for a practitioner/teacher role. Although the preparation of the practitioner has not been singled out into a discrete chapter, the reader will not find it difficult to see that the primary focus of the entire curriculum is the development of this role. The reader may also find it useful to reread portions of Miller's chapter in Part I of this book, which pertain to her function as a teacher of advanced practitioners.

Readers interested in analyzing and refining their own roles will find the method described by Klassen and DiMotto an interesting and useful guide, irrespective of the role in which they function. The detail provided is also for the benefit of educators who are as yet unfamiliar with the potential of a role development course.

Dr. Wallenborn can rightfully be called "the teacher's teacher." Her chapter on the preparation of practitioners as educators will help neophyte teachers to gain insight into many facets of a faculty role. Graduate program faculty should find the process and content description of the teaching component a valuable resource not just for developing a teaching component but for evaluating and refining other components in the program.

The chapter by Goodyear was written toward the completion of her Master's program while she was still a student. Since graduation, she has been working as a practitioner/teacher on a rehabilitation unit through a joint appointment between Marquette University and a local hospital. The reader will note that at this stage of development there is no apparent focus on the research aspect of the role. This is in keeping with the progression and perception of the role as referred to in the Introductions to Part I and Part II of this book.

The final section of Wallenborn's chapter on a proposed post-master's program for teachers of nursing demonstrates an interdisciplinary effort initiated by nurse educators. The potential benefit of such a program for nurse educators in both academic and service settings is obvious and is in no way intended as an equivalent of or competition for a doctorate in nursing. For nurse educators who have never had the benefit of a course in curriculum development, the process described can improve your understanding of this faculty function.

This book would not be complete without emphasizing the importance of continuing education in the development of practitioner/teachers. The final chapter, therefore, looks at existing and potential types of continuing education courses that can help nurse educators develop a full faculty role or a full inservice educator role.

9
Developing a Role-Oriented Model for Graduate Education

Lorraine Machan

One of the major problems of graduate education for professional nurses has been the failure to provide adequate and flexible role preparation. The fact is that while nursing as a professional discipline must provide graduate education that strengthens the practice of nursing, many of these graduates prepared as advanced practitioners accept employment as teachers of nursing or administrators with little or no preparation for the roles of teacher or administrator. In addition, as stated by Dorothy A. Mereness, "there seems to be little consensus as to the essential content which should be included in postbaccalaureate education."[1] Recent references to sources expressing concern are the Nahm report to the New England Board of Higher Education, a National League for Nursing Paper published in July 1975, and the McLane study which has a well-documented review of literature indicative of the need for nurse educators to concern themselves with competencies that all graduates of higher degrees in nursing should possess.[2]

Christman has described the full professional role as encompassing "the subrole segments of service, education, consultation and research."[3] It becomes evident that there are core behaviors associated with these broad categories which are essential to fulfilling these subroles in *any* profession. An education which is role-oriented must not only provide content for a necessary knowledge base, but must provide the student with the opportunities and techniques to develop desirable behavior patterns. The question that arises is who decides what patterns of behavior are desirable and undesirable. "Unless there is a consensus and clarity of the norms, values and behaviors expected within the given profession, it will be increasingly difficult to socialize the neophyte into its ranks."[4]

Faculty members involved with the master's program in nursing at Marquette University have been interested in role concepts for over 10 years, and it was this group interest that laid a foundation for the McLane study "Core Competencies of Master's Prepared Nurses and Implication for Program Development" referred to above. This study identified a core of 25 competencies that all Master's prepared graduates are expected to attain, irrespective of the specific role in which they would function—practitioner, teacher, or manager. In addition, the study identified some expected role-specific competencies.

With the aid of a three-year grant (1976-1979) from the Division of Nursing of the Department of Health, Education and Welfare, the faculty expanded the concepts of the role-oriented model it implemented in Fall 1975 (Fig. 9.1) The McLane study competencies were utilized as one basis for program evaluation.

For purpose of analysis, the faculty conceptualized the components of the roles, practitioner, teacher and manager separately. However, in implementing the curriculum some learning experiences provide for the development of common role components while others provide for development of components specific to practitioner, teacher, or manager role (see Fig. 9.2) It is interesting to note that the original identification of specific role components stimulated lengthy discussions that led to a list of eleven common role components and less than half as many role-specific components. Preparation for the multifaceted roles of practitioner/teacher and practitioner/manager is achieved through identification of role components and behaviors, design of courses providing learning opportunities for developing the behaviors, and through the unique, self-directed, and continuously evolving combination of components and behaviors within the student. The process used in developing the objectives and critical indicators for the teaching component is described in the chapter by Wallenborn. This same process was and is used in developing objectives and critical indicators for other program components. At the beginning of a course, student attention is focused on the role behaviors and critical indicators and the level objectives for which the particular course provides learning opportunities. Level objectives for the Care of the Adult option based on total program objectives are shown in Table 9.1.

The program has a strong clinical focus. Students admitted are expected to have developed physical assessment and basic nursing assessment skills before admission to the program, or if they have deficits to remove them before admission to the first clinical nursing course. Students are also expected to have had a reasonable amount of postbaccalaureate practice experience in the area of their option (adult or child). Each of these options has two four-credit nursing courses with practicums of 6 to 10 hours per week. A nursing theories course is a prerequisite to the clinical courses.

Students in the Care of the Adult option are primary care givers to a case

MODEL FOR A ROLE-ORIENTED CURRICULUM PREPARING

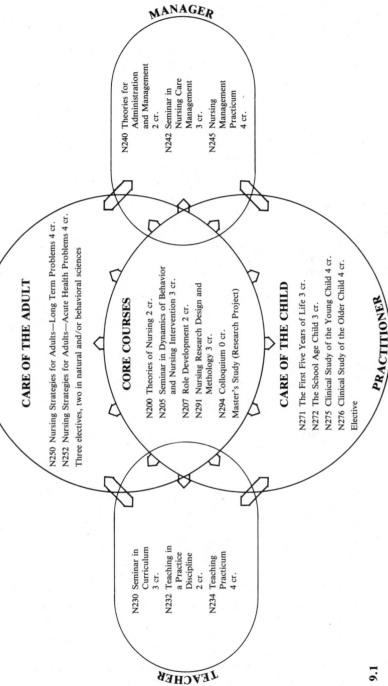

MANAGER

N240 Theories for Administration and Management 2 cr.

N242 Seminar in Nursing Care Management 3 cr.

N245 Nursing Management Practicum 4 cr.

PRACTITIONER/MANAGER

PRACTITIONER

PRACTITIONER/TEACHER

CARE OF THE ADULT

N250 Nursing Strategies for Adults—Long Term Problems 4 cr.

N252 Nursing Strategies for Adults—Acute Health Problems 4 cr.

Three electives, two in natural and/or behavioral sciences

CORE COURSES

N200 Theories of Nursing 2 cr.

N205 Seminar in Dynamics of Behavior and Nursing Intervention 3 cr.

N207 Role Development 2 cr.

N291 Nursing Research Design and Methology 3 cr.

N294 Colloquium 0 cr.

Master's Study (Research Project)

CARE OF THE CHILD

N271 The First Five Years of Life 3 cr.

N272 The School Age Child 3 cr.

N275 Clinical Study of the Young Child 4 cr.

N276 Clinical Study of the Older Child 4 cr.

Elective

PRACTITIONER

N230 Seminar in Curriculum 3 cr.

N232 Teaching in a Practice Discipline 2 cr.

N234 Teaching Practicum 4 cr.

TEACHER

Fig. 9.1

COMMON AND SPECIFIC ROLE COMPONENTS FOR PRACTITIONER/TEACHER AND MANAGER

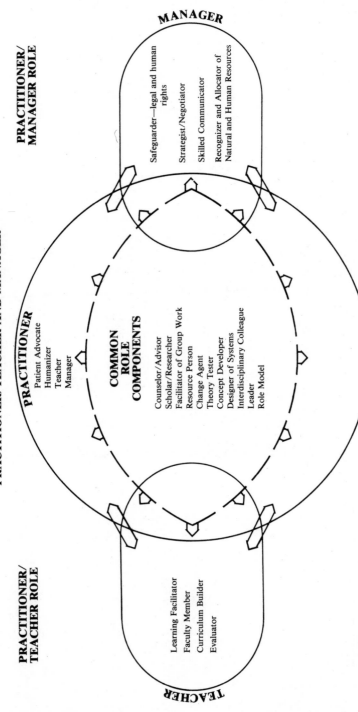

**PRACTITIONER/
MANAGER ROLE**

MANAGER

Safeguarder—legal and human
rights

Strategist/Negotiator

Skilled Communicator

Recognizer and Allocator of
Natural and Human Resources

PRACTITIONER

Patient Advocate
Humanizer
Teacher
Manager

**COMMON
ROLE
COMPONENTS**

Counselor/Advisor
Scholar/Researcher
Facilitator of Group Work
Resource Person
Change Agent
Theory Tester
Concept Developer
Designer of Systems
Interdisciplinary Colleague
Leader
Role Model

**PRACTITIONER/
TEACHER ROLE**

Learning Facilitator
Faculty Member
Curriculum Builder
Evaluator

TEACHER

Fig. 9.2

Table 9.1   Level Objectives for the Care of the Adult Option in a Graduate Program in Nursing

Level I	Level II	Level III — Terminal Objectives for Care of Adult
Graduate Program Objective No. 1:	Command of a body of knowledge relevant to the health care of a specific group of clients.	
Knows concepts and research applicable to adults who are chronically ill.	Knows critical research relevant to nursing cares of selected adult clients with acute health problems.	Utilizes analytic skills and research processes to identify adult client problems and nursing strategies that contribute to the body of nursing knowledge.
Select and utilize concepts and theories from biopsycho-social sciences to expand the foundation for nursing practice.	Utilize research methodology to identify nursing problems and make contributions to nursing's body of knowledge.	
Utilize knowledge of the dynamics of behavior of individuals and families in achieving health results.		
Graduate Program Objective No. 2:	Ability to test theories derived from existing bodies of knowledge and the study of a specific group of clients.	
Utilize theories from bio-psychosocial sciences in providing nursing care.	Use and/or develop a specific theoretical matrix for making observations and formu-lating clinical hunches.	Identifies and tests concepts and theories derived from the nursing and biopsychosocial sciences and own nursing practice.

Table 9.1—Continued

Level I	Level II	Level III — Terminal Objectives for Care of Adult
Demonstrates skill in formulating predictive principles to design nursing strategies.	Develop and test hypotheses relative to own nursing practice.	
	Formulate new concepts relative to client and family responses to illness.	
Graduate Program Objective No: 3:	Ability to utilize a conceptual framework as a guide for nursing practice, management and teaching nursing consistent with a holistic view of man and a changing society.	
Adopts a conceptual framework for own nursing practice congruent with own beliefs and values.	Further evolves a conceptual framework for nursing congruent with own beliefs and values.	Engages in nursing practice which reflects the critical use of a conceptual framework for nursing.
Knows basic families of nursing theories (e.g., adaptation, self-care, behavioral systems, interactional models).	Tests selected aspects of nursing frameworks to determine their effect on perception of client problems and nursing interventions.	
Conceptualizes nursing and defines the scope of nursing practice congruent with a holistic view of man.		
Graduate Program Objective No. 4:	Ability to improve nursing practice, management or teaching through the utilization of the research process.	

Systematically applies research findings to a selected client group.

Utilizes disciplined data collection in building a personal repertoire of nursing behaviors.

Utilizes the research process and research findings to describe, explain, and predict nursing practice.

Becomes sensitized to problem areas in nursing needing systematic investigation.

Critically evaluates the use of research findings in the solution of clinical problems.

Formulates and challenges conclusions of clinical studies done by self and others.

Graduate Program Objective No. 5: Ability to utilize deliberate decision-making to select and implement strategies to yield predictable outcomes.

Arrives at statements of nursing problems deducted from the student's adopted conceptual framework.

Conceptualizes nursing diagnoses which contribute to the typology of nursing diagnoses.

Formulates nursing diagnoses and utilizes practice and research-based nursing strategies.

Designs unique and specific nursing interventions relative to the formulated nursing diagnosis.

Prescribes and implements nursing actions based on research and/or hypotheses derived from supportive sciences and practice.

Graduate Program Objective No. 6: Ability to develop, test, and apply sets of criteria for the purpose of assessing outcomes achieved through nursing care.

Develops a set of nursing outcome criteria for a specific patient.

Develops and tests with clients and peers sets of nursing outcome criteria for patient problems common to a selected client group.

Develops, tests, and applies sets of criteria to determine whether nursing contributed to holistic man's ability to care for himself on a continuing basis.

Table 9.1—Continued

Level I	Level II	Level III — Terminal Objectives for Care of Adult
Graduate Program Objective No. 7:	Ability to initiate, maintain and promote intra-and inter-disciplinary colleagueship in providing health care.	
Initiates relationships with individuals in own and other disciplines to locate resources within the health care system to help clients achieve health results.	Makes prospective decisions about health care in collaboration with client and health professionals.	Develops skills in interdisciplinary collaboration for the purpose of planning and implementing programs for adults with specific problems.
Graduate Program Objective No. 8:	Ability to design programs for nursing care, education, and research.	
Analyzes the health care system to determine the needs for program for a specific group of clients.	Initiates and participates in planning and implementing needed health care services for specific groups of clients.	Designs, implements, and evaluates programs to provide clients with special skills which enhance their self-care agency.
Identifies conditions within a health care agency which facilitate or inhibit the designing of programs to meet the needs of clients.		
Graduate Program Objective No. 9:	Competence for and socialization to the roles of advanced practitioner and beginning teacher of nursing or advanced practitioner and manager of nursing.	

Communicates a concept of nursing to consumers, peers, and other health workers.

Exhibits role model behavior for students and health workers.

Articulates a future-focused role image.

Demonstrates professional competence and socialization for the role of advanced practitioner.

Graduate Program Objective No. 10:

Those personal characteristics appropriate for the advanced professional practitioner and the beginning teacher of nursing or the advanced professional practitioner and manager of nursing.

Has a commitment to professional excellence.

Contributes to humanizing environment.

Creates a climate conducive to potentiating self-actualiza-tion and professional excellence.

Demonstrates growth in inter-personal competence.

Develops colleague relationships with faculty and other profes-sionals.

load of patients they carry throughout the semester. They define the case load by the area of their own choice. For some this is in traditional medical, surgical nursing classification. For others it is in terms of concepts such as nursing diagnosis, compliance, stress patterns, coping behaviors, developmental needs. Though the curriculum organization may appear to be rigid, there is flexibility within the courses. Whatever the defined case load, the student uses the same defined population type for both nursing practicums. Within limits, the institutional setting is also in line with student choice. If it is in a setting other than the one in which the instructor usually works with students, a master's prepared preceptor must be available as a resource person and to assist in evaluating the student as an advanced practitioner.

Table 9.2 shows the Care of the Adult, Practitioner Component objectives and critical indicators placed in the format of the student evaluation tool now being tested for validity. The tool is used in both practicum courses but the levels of expectation for achievement are different. Student and preceptor evaluate independently. The form to be completed by the preceptor differs from Table 9.2 only in that the preceptor is directed to rate the student. The ratings and comments are tabulated in preceptor/student pairs and reviewed by faculty in an effort to determine validity. Through this process the tool has undergone two revisions and evaluation of it will continue on a yearly basis.

If the faculty has not developed research skills to the level of professional expectation it is unlikely that many of the students will emerge as graduates with the skills. ". . . nursing research must be integrated and its values institutionalized within graduate programs and not merely treated as embellishment to the College's other educational efforts and offerings."[5] To help students assimilate the concept that research is an inherent part of nursing practice, faculty members in the Care of the Adult option designed long-term research projects within broad areas discussed in the clinical nursing courses and upon which the student focuses in the practice that is a requirement for both courses. These have included studies on nursing diagnoses, coping strategies, self esteem in the chronically ill, stress, humanizing factors, pain, and studies on families of patients suffering heart attacks. Students contribute observations to a data pool and some of them have been involved in data analysis and interpretation. Miller describes this in greater detail in Part I of this book. She also writes about the effect of her practice and research role on students and faculty colleagues.

Students have a course in research design and method, and a research project carried out and written up as a master's study (essay or thesis) is a degree requirement. A weekly nursing research colloquium was introduced when the curriculum was implemented to stimulate research interest and provide an opportunity for students, faculty, and professionals from the community to discuss completed or ongoing projects. The growth in nurs-

Table 9.2   Graduate Program of Studies—Care of the Adult Component
FINAL EVALUATION FORM To be completed by master student

DIRECTIONS: The objectives for the Care of the Adult component are listed at the top of each section (I-IV). Critical indicators are included beneath each objective. You are asked to rate yourself by circling the most appropriate symbol. They are as follows: WP-well prepared; AP-adequately prepared; NI-needs improvement; NO-No opportunity to observe.

In the space provided at the right of the paper, give an example of an incident or behavior that would help us determine why you rated yourself as you did. Not all items necessarily apply to every student practicum setting.

Objectives					Comments/Examples
I. Utilize analytic skills and research processes to identify adult client* problems and to design nursing strategies that contribute both to the well-being of the client and to the body of nursing knowledge					
A. Consistently validate with client assessment of his health state, pattern of coping, and ability to seek and utilize resources	WP	AP	NI	NO	
B. Conceptualize and classify client vulnerabilities and responses to health-illness	WP	AP	NI	NO	
C. Derive concepts for own practice from biopsychosocial and nursing science	WP	AP	NI	NO	

Table 9.2—Continued

Objectives	WP	AP	NI	NO	Comments/Examples
D. Design plans of care with clients to meet their current and emerging health needs	WP	AP	NI	NO	
II. Utilize the research process and research findings to describe, explain, predict and prescribe nursing practice, adding to the body of objective knowledge					
A. Identify problem areas in nursing care of adults needing systematic investigation	WP	AP	NI	NO	
B. Articulate and investigate own concerns, questions and problems utilizing appropriate research process	WP	AP	NI	NO	
C. Refine nursing practice through clinical research	WP	AP	NI	NO	
D. Communicate research findings	WP	AP	NI	NO	
III. Engages in nursing practice which reflects the critical use of a concept of nursing and incorporates an ethical basis for decision-making					

A. Utilize interpersonal and family theories in the establishment and maintenance of helping relationships

WP	AP	NI	NO

B. Design and implement programs of nursing based on nursing practice theories

WP	AP	NI	NO

C. Utilize disciplined data collection in building a personal repertoire of nursing behavior

WP	AP	NI	NO

D. Develop and apply criteria to evaluate the content, process and outcomes of own practice consistent with professional ethics and standards

WP	AP	NI	NO

IV. Demonstrate personal and professional growth toward socialization to the role of advanced practitioner

A. Initiate collaboration with interdisciplinary and intradisciplinary colleagues to plan and implement programs of care for adults with special problems

WP	AP	NI	NO

Table 9.2—Continued

Objectives					Comments/Examples
B. Demonstrate the independent function of the nurse in the counseling role	WP	AP	NI	NO	
C. Design, implement, and evaluate planned change in the practice setting	WP	AP	NI	NO	
D. Create a climate conducive to potentiating the self-actualization and professional excellence of others	WP	AP	NI	NO	
E. Evaluate for nursing practice the significance of current issues and trends relevant to health care	WP	AP	NI	NO	

*The term client refers to individuals, families, groups seeking and/or utilizing resources to improve their health status.

ing research has been reflected in the Colloquium schedules and in faculty and student or graduate publications.

The core courses, Dynamics of Behavior and Nursing Intervention and Role Development, both are designed to assist students in development of their role as either practitioner/teacher or practitioner/manager, the former course focusing on the counseling role and the latter on the role development process.

Role Development, a two-credit course, is taken concurrently with a nursing practicum (preferably the first clinical course) or with either the teaching or management practicum. The content is limited to reading and discussion in the areas of role theory, systems theory, and change theory. Students keep a journal or log of their role development process. (See the following chapter in this book.) Students are introduced to four models at the beginning of the course, which give direction and definition to the role implementation log. These models are the frameworks by Kahn and Quinn, Aradine and Denyes, Kramer and Schmalenberg, and Filley.[6]

PROGRAM EVALUATION

Course and teacher evaluation are university expectations at this institution. In addition to the University form in use, some nursing faculty members have designed supplemental evaluation forms which they request students to complete. Total program evaluation is carried out both by the University Graduate School office and the College of Nursing.

Table 9.3 shows an evaluation of the present program objectives by graduates of the program who had received their degree at least six months prior to evaluating. The majority of ratings fall in the first two categories. Although the rating of 5 was given by only one graduate to objective 10, three additional individuals indicated by comments the need for clarification or revision of this objective. The form sent to graduates asked for additional comments. These have not been included because of difficulty in preserving anonymity. However, the cooperation received from graduates and expressions of satisfaction and constructive criticism are encouraging. Although the majority of graduates are employed in either teaching or practice functions, there is a trend developing for graduates of this program to seek employment in the practitioner/teacher role. Also there is evidence of a few graduates putting role components together into new combinations to form innovative roles which they are developing for themselves. One graduate directed her program development as a student to a role as a thanatologist, and is now functioning as a clinical specialist in thanatology.

"We have the opportunity to proceed as Nightingale advocated: as self-directed professionals, defining our own functions and roles and making

Table 9.3 Evaluation of Objectives for a Role-Oriented Graduate Program

Name _____   Date Graduated _____

Date Entered Program _____

Option: Practitioner/Teacher _____   Care of the Adult _____
        Practitioner/Manager _____   Care of the Child _____

Present Position:

Please rate each objective by circling the appropriate number on a scale from 1 to 5, interpreted as follows:

1. Realistic; reflects the usual nature of my practice.
2. Realistic; I meet this objective often in my work.
3. Realistic as a program objective, but I am seldom able to apply it in my present position.
4. Realistic as a program objective, but I am never able to apply it in my present position.
5. Unrealistic; the program did not prepare me to meet this objective.

Objectives	Rating Scale	Comments
Objective 1. The graduate of the program is expected to demonstrate command of a body of knowledge relevant to the health care of a specific group of clients.	1 2 3 4 5 ———————— 8 5 1 1 2	Worked with renal failure and transplant patient in school. Now working with totally different client group. My clinical experience prior to graduate school enabled me to meet this objective successfully. Without a strong clinical background an individual would probably experience difficulty meeting this objective with

only graduate school clinical experience. I learned many more general nursing concepts in depth that can be applied to many client groups.

The client group with whom I worked in graduate school is not the same that I am working with now. Expertise with the first group taught me how to specialize, how to research a client group in practice and the literature and gave me confidence in myself as an expert in at least one field.

It is imperative that I be informed of the psychologic as well as the psychosocial aspects of care for the terminally ill and bereaved.

The freedom to do this in the program is great. The ability to fulfill the objective varies with the group of patients on the hospital unit at any one time. If there are patients representative of the specific group, the objective is usually met.

	1	2	3	4	5
	5	7	2	1	1

Objective 2. The graduate of the program is expected to demonstrate ability to test theories derived from existing bodies of knowledge and the study of a specific group of clients.

Use self-care theory daily.

I find I must constantly focus on this to prevent myself from becoming stagnant.

The field is new thus theories must be tested and often revised.

Very applicable to nursing today. Difficult to do with any consistency in a part time teaching position on a general medsurg unit.

I'll keep working on it though! Lack of time is a factor.

Table 9.3—Continued

Objectives	Rating Scale					Comments
	1	2	3	4	5	
Objective 3. The graduate of the program is expected to demonstrate ability to utilize a conceptual framework as a guide for nursing practice, management and teaching nursing consistent with a holistic view of man and a changing society.	10	5			2	Especially helpful. Many advanced concepts were taught that fit into a conceptual framework chosen by the student —but advanced concepts related to physiologic man are weak as compared to other aspects of man unless the student designs her own learning experiences.
						I feel MU strongly emphasized this. Thank God we were presented with a variety of theories, because there are instances when I see value in relating to one rather than another, depending on the situation.
						Roy works quite well for me along with a combination of thanatological models.
						I found this objective quite possible to accomplish, facilitated by the working environment within the MUCN faculty.
Objective 4. The graduate of the program is expected to demonstrate ability to improve nursing practice, management or teaching through the utilization of the research process.	3	7	5	1	1	Research course should have students doing miniresearch projects; otherwise our essay or thesis is the only (massive) study completed.
						Research is ongoing in my practice based on the documentation of care within the Kinlein Theory of care. I utilize clinical research on a limited basis in the nursing setting to demonstrate theories to nursing staff. Research does not seem to be a high priority in most institutional settings. Our highly developed quality assurance program allows us to do this on a sophisticated level, but I am often able to find opportunities in every day practice to utilize a research process.

Too heavy a faculty load to become involved in as much research as I'd like to be.

The strong research focus is the main benefit of the program.

Objective 5. The graduate of the program is expected to demonstrate ability to utilize deliberate decision-making to select and implement strategies to yield predictable outcomes.

1	2	3	4	5
12	1	1	1	2

This is dependent on the institutional setting but I would hope a graduate of any accredited nursing program would be able to meet this objective. N207 did present these concepts well, but there are times when the situations within the 'real' world are still rather startling, and objective thinking is not automatic for me.

This is vital to masters level practice and is helped by the research component. The program prepared us well for this. I personally have difficulty with this one.

Not the program's drawback—I just have a hard time making up my mind.

Objective 6. The graduate of the program is expected to demonstrate ability to develop, test, and apply sets of criteria for the purpose of assessing outcomes achieved through nursing care.

1	2	3	4	5
8	3	1	2	2

I teach a course in QA.

Again relating to our QA program, this makes it easier for me to incorporate this heavily.

However, I don't think my preparation in this area is due to the graduate program.

The program prepared us well for this. My background in this is shaky—however my program was somewhat unusual and not representative of the 1976–77 curriculum. This could be stressed more in the program since it is so crucial in nursing today.

Objective 7. The graduate of the program is expected to demonstrate ability to initiate, maintain and promote intra- and interdisciplinary colleagueship in providing health care.

1	2	3	4	5
12	1	2		2

The program prepared us well for this.

As a masters level practitioner, the staff looks constantly to me for help with this.

Table 9.3—Continued

Objectives	Rating Scale					Comments
	1	2	3	4	5	Consistently interpreting the changing role of nursing to RN's, MD's, LPN's public. I believe that much of one's ability in this area is related to what the persons brought to the program as opposed to what they got from the program.
Objective 8. The graduate of the program is expected to demonstrate ability to design programs for nursing care, education and research.	7	7	1	2		Within my job, I not only design patient teaching experiences for staff nurses, but also learning experience for staff nurses. The graduate program, I felt, did foster creativity and effectiveness in organization so as to achieve designated outcomes. I am able to apply this because U is currently involved in a total curriculum change. I did feel competent in my position as 1 of 6 faculty members chosen to plan and articulate this new curriculum. I have just been promoted to this position. However, my objectives include exploration of the feasibility of the practice lab being used for research and continuing education needs. Feel well prepared considering brief amount of time in graduate school.
Objective 9. The graduate of the program is expected to demonstrate competence for and socialization to the roles of advanced practitioner and beginning teacher of nursing or advanced practitioner and manager of nursing.	1	2	3	4	5	Successful due to prior experience and background in nursing. Although we did spend time in graduate school considering socialization into advance practice, I think it is almost always an overwhelming and at times devastating experience.
	11	4		2		

Objective 10. The graduate of the program is expected to demonstrate those personal characteristics appropriate for the advanced professional practitioner and the beginning teacher of nursing or the advanced professional practitioner and manager of nursing.

1	2	3	4	5
			13	1

Personal growth has preceded my professional development in practice.

Graduate education at MU has facilitated this process. This objective is nebulous and impossible to measure. Personal characteristics may or may not be influenced by the graduate school program.

My personal characteristics were altered little by graduate school attendance and are based on a total life experience that is in perpetual evolution.

I'm not sure of the meaning of this objective and cannot evaluate it. I can honestly state that across the board the people in my peer group left the program with a great deal more "professional characteristics" than what we came with.

This seems to be the best learned once in the field—systems theory is vital to this. Perhaps "those personal characteristics" should be clarified. Not sure exactly what is meant.

ADDITIONAL COMMENTS

our own decisions and assessments. . . . It is presently our opportunity and our challenge to define new roles to meet society's changing needs and to extend our own theories."[7] If the program has been the role-oriented model intended, its value will be evident for many years to come for the graduates will have learned strategies to adapt to and even create the new roles that changes in society will demand.

REFERENCES

1. Mereness, Dorothy A.: Graduate education as one dean sees it. *Nursing Outlook,* 23:638–641, October 1975.
2. Nahm, Helen: Graduate education in nursing in New England. Wellesley, Mass., A Report to the New England Board of Higher Education, June 1975; Lodge, Mary P.: *Facts and Reflections about Masters Education in Nursing in the United States.* New York, National League for Nursing, 1975; McLane, Audrey M.: Core competencies of master's prepared nurses and implications for program development. Ph.D. Dissertation, Marquette University, 1975; McLane, Audrey M.: Core competencies of master's prepared nurses. *Nursing Research,* 27:48–53, January 1978.
3. Christman, Luther: The practitioner-teacher: A working paper. Rush-Presbyterian-St. Luke's Medical Center, Chicago, December, 1973. (A working document for faculty deliberation. By personal communication.); Christman, Luther: The autonomous staff in the hospital. Paper delivered at A.N.A Convention under the auspices of the National Joint Practice Commission, Atlantic City, June 9, 1976.
4. Lum, Jean L. J.: Reference Groups and Professional Socialization. In Hardy, Margaret and Conway, Mary (eds.): *Role Theory.* New York, Appleton-Century-Crofts, 1978.
5. Cleland, Virginia: Nursing Research and Graduate Education. *Nursing Outlook,* 23:642–645, 1975.
6. Kahn, Robert and Quinn, Robert: *Role Stress: A Framework for Analysis.* In McLean, Alan (ed.): *Mental Health and Work Organizations.* Chicago, Rand McNally and Co., 1970; Aradine, Carolyn and Denyes, Mary Jean: Activities and pressures of clinical nurse specialists. *Nursing Research,* 21:411–418, September-October 1972; Kramer, Marlene and Schmalenberg, Claudia E.: Conflict: The cutting edge of growth. *Journal of Nursing Administration,* 6:19–25, October 1976; Filley, Alan: *Interpersonal Conflict Resolution.* Glenview, IL, Scott, Foresman and Co., 1975.
7. Walsh, Margaret E.: Planning for the future—nursing's role. In *Health Care in the 1980s.* New York, National League for Nursing, Publ. No. 52-1755, 1979, pp. 12–31.

10
Utilization of the Log as a Teaching Tool in a Role-Development Course

Loretta Klassen and Jean Wouters DiMotto

A graduate curriculum based on a role-oriented model implies a significant focus on process as content. Role Development, a core course within this curriculum, helps students in the process of role development through the analysis of relevant interactions evolving from the concurrent practicum experience of a practitioner, teacher, or manager function.

The current course evolved over a three-year period. At a very early phase of its development, it became clear that a student log or journal would be valuable in evaluating the student's progress in role development. Initially, this was tested at the end of the semester by two independently prepared summaries of direct quotes from student logs, indicating achievement of each course objective. One summary was prepared by the course instructor and the other by a faculty member who had audited the course. Privacy was maintained by identifying students by number rather than name. Also, neither faculty member was involved with the graduate students in any of the areas reflected in the log.

These two summaries were compared to determine the extent of agreement. As a result of this, and with student input either in terminal or ongoing conferences, it became apparent that more structure was necessary to provide a more objective means of evaluating the role process documented in the logs. Two changes were made in the course: (1) objectives that were not meaningful and relevant, as evidenced by lack of documentation in the log, were revised, and (2) four models were introduced early in the course to give students a framework for developing their logs.[1] These models helped students to ask themselves the right questions when documenting their progress.

Using the Kahn and Quinn framework, instructor and students were able to pose a number of questions significant to role development:

1. Are communication processes from significant individuals in the professional environment to the student prescriptive or evaluative? What is the significance of this?
2. What inadequacies exist in the pattern of role expectations?
3. What inadequacies are there in personal resources which help the person comply with role expectations?
4. What was the perceptual cognitive response in a stress situation?
5. What coping mechanisms were utilized by the student?
6. What system influences were evident?

The second model from Aradine and Denyes introduced the grouping of categories in examining role pressures. This gave rise to the following considerations:

1. Use of these four categories in rating role pressures (self-pressure, system pressure, role pressure, other pressure)
2. Changes in role pressure over a period of time
3. Examination of cause and effect of role pressures

The third and fourth models, Kramer and Schmalenberg, and Filley, stimulated students to examine their approaches to resolving conflicts, decision making, and coping strategies.

Clarification of course objectives and use of the four models enhanced subsequent development of behavioral characteristics. These critical behaviors facilitate the instructor's and student's identification of meaningful cues in the log, thereby providing the opportunity for adequate feedback while the process is taking place.

Another outcome of the review activity and course revision was identification of significant patterns or themes in the log which provide insight into the role development process and content for class discussion. The behavioral characteristics were placed in the format of an evaluation tool (See Table 10.1) with the goal that both instructor and student document progress throughout the semester. During the extended process of deriving these behavioral characteristics through log review, it became apparent that the clearer and more refined behavioral indices became, the better students were able to analyze and document their role development. From 24 student logs (Spring semester '78, Spring semester '79) explored in depth, the following four patterns emerged: (1) change of role pressures over the semester, (2) the problem-solving approach became the major method of conflict resolution, (3) doctor-nurse conflicts were frequent, and (4) reintegration of self took place by the end of the semester.

Table 10.1   Evaluation Tool for Role Implementation Log

Directions: On the basis of the student log, change project, and discussion this semester in Role Development, rate student's performance based on the following guide:

Guide: **1** little progress observed or documented.
2 moderate progress observed or documented.
3 high level of progress observed or documented.
NO not observed or documented.

Objectives: Course objectives are based on three content areas:
Role Theory, Systems Theory, and Change Theory.

Objectives: Role Theory: Student is able to:
1. Utilize an understanding or behavior while incorporating the role of practitioner/teacher or practitioner/manager
2. Utilize the concept of identity while incorporating the role of practitioner/teacher or practitioner/manager.
3. Analyze factors which positively or inversely influence the role transition taking place as practitioner/teacher or practitioner/manager.
4. Create and test role conflict reducing strategies.

Examples of Behavioral Characteristics in this Area would include:	Progress Rating	Documentation or Comments
1. Identifies communication processes from role set to focal person as prescriptive or evaluative and determines significance	1 2 3 NO	
2. Identifies existence and nature of role conflict or ambiguity	1 2 3 NO	
3. Examines nature of personal resources and reflexive role expectations of the focal person	1 2 3 NO	
4. Determines alteration of perceptual-cognitive responses in a stress situation	1 2 3 NO	

Table 10.1—Continued

Examples of Behavioral Characteristics in this Area would include:	Progress Rating	Documentation or Comments
5. Analyzes coping mechanisms utilized in role conflict or stress	1 2 3 NO	
6. Evaluates changes in cause and effect of role pressures over the semester	1 2 3 NO	
7. Identifies nature of role facilitators	1 2 3 NO	

Objectives: Systems Theory: Student is able to:
1. Identify the properties of an open system
2. Analyze the organization and interaction-influence systems in complex health care organizations

Examples of Behavioral Characteristics in this Area would include:	Progress Rating	Documentation or Comments
1. Demonstrates awareness of the influence of organizations on the role set as this relates to focal person	1 2 3 NO	
2. Applies understanding of properties of an open system at an operational level	1 2 3 NO	
3. Identifies conflicts related to differences of values of the role set as compared to focal person		

Objectives: Change Theory: Student is able to:
          1. Analyze the process of change within a professional setting
          2. Design, implement, and evaluate planned change in a particular setting

Examples of Behavioral Characteristics in this Area would include:	Progress Rating	Documentation or Comments
1. Shows evidence of functioning as a change agent	1 2 3 NO	
2. Demonstrates awareness of process of change within the open system	1 2 3 NO	
3. Identifies strategies utilized in a change process	1 2 3 NO	
4. Synthesizes theories of change in the change project	1 2 3 NO	
5. Selects legitimate focus for change project	1 2 3 NO	
6. Supports change project with relevant data	1 2 3 NO	

CHANGE OF ROLE PRESSURES

The first pattern, change of role pressures over the semester, was frequently documented in the logs. Initial conflicts expressed in the logs reflected concerns over discrepancies between self-expectations and personal resources, or self-expectations and expectations of role senders.[2] One study concerning clinical nurse specialists stated that the most frequently identified pressures among four groupings (self, role, system, others) were self pressures, i.e., difficulty setting priorities, self expectations too high, loneliness and isolation, and expectations were too diversified.[3] Later, the focus of the logs seemed to reflect discrepancies between system and environment. A representative sampling from logs reflects this transition of conflicts over the semester. Both of the students cited were developing a practitioner role.

2/5   Monday, first day in ICU . . . I was nervous about seeing a patient in ICU for two reasons, both involving expectations. I was not certain that the head nurse in ICU understood why I was choosing the particular patient and what I would take responsibility for—possibly components of role ambiguity. Secondly, I was not certain of my own reflexive role expectations. When I reflected on the role I intended to take, that of advanced practitioner, I felt conflict involving the expectation of the role senders [Kahn and Quinn 1970] (in this case the head nurse and preceptor) and my personal resources. Assessing the client in behavioral, emotional, and environmental terms is a resource I have. Assessing the client in depth physiologically I am unable to do and am not certain how much I should pursue this skill.

2/18   My client had been moved to intermediate care and was progressing well . . . I had begun teaching . . . the family viewed me as a helper and offered evaluative feedback.

3/6   Evaluation of Role Implementation to date: Most of the stress involved thus far has focused around my reflexive expectations and being able to meet these expectations. The second area that has contributed to my stress is the environment—the empirical model—within the system. Although I feel I'm following the rules of the game, the staff has another set that I am just beginning to learn. I am beginning to feel somewhat more at ease, especially after relating the teaching plan difficulty and seeing a change. The role of advanced practitioner so far seems lonely.

4/14   To date I'm satisfied with my role development. Nurses on the floor where the majority of my clients were seemed to realize I have some clinical competence. All of the team leaders discussed my clients with me and attempted to gain knowledge from the theories and concepts I used.

In contrast, the following student reflects similar initial pressures, but was less advanced in the graduate program and expresses perhaps a higher level of anxiety which is somewhat representative of the beginning graduate student.

1/30   My role! What really is my role? I wish I knew. Right now I'm in limbo. I have no clear-cut definition of what my role should be or is now. Sometimes I'm a graduate student; sometimes a staff nurse . . . right now I'm not even sure how I'll find the clinical area in which I'll practice. I haven't toured it and I know very few people at that institution. What if they don't help me? What if I don't know what to do? What if everything I do turns out wrong? What exactly am I going to do anyway? That I am suffering from a classic case of expectation-generated stress does not make the symptoms any less painful.

2/14   For the first time since I started, I almost feel as though I have some sense of direction. My one patient is improving and I feel more comfortable in some aspects of what I am doing. I can also begin to see some development of strengths. Tonight I approached and interacted with the family of a patient I hope to contract with tomorrow (she was in surgery at the time). While this doesn't sound very earth-shattering, it really was a step for me in this new role.

4/19   I now feel I've had to work very hard to change from being primarily a "doer" to a real "helper." My work as a staff nurse has been primarily as a "doer" first and "helper," if there was time. By "helper" I mean someone who was able to help the patient in all spheres, not just do the necessary tasks required to stabilize a patient physiologically. When I entered a situation where the patients were fairly stable physiologically and I did not have to do something first, it was difficult at first . . . to determine the area where help was needed and then to convey my helpfulness. Now I can see, after reading and learning from others, how much I have improved.

This student was coping with the initial socialization process of a graduate student in addition to the role development of advanced practitioner. In comparison, the first student indicated a rapid transition of role pressures. This might be attributed to a more advanced standing in the graduate program and condensed experiential learning in graduate school, where accelerated growth takes place.

PROBLEM-SOLVING TO RESOLVE CONFLICT

A second pattern frequently reflected in student logs was problem solving as a predominant method of conflict resolution.

The individual subjected to stress will attempt to utilize personal resources and problem-solving processes to manage the environment and reduce role strain. If the negative experience—strain—is not reduced, there is reason to assume that other adaptive responses may be employed.[4]

Hardy then goes on to state that strain-reducing strategies may range from simple problem-solving methods, through various bargaining techniques, to symbolic interaction strategies.

In the evaluation of logs, there was very little evidence of strategies utilized beyond the problem-solving approach. Is this because nurses are socialized in the nursing process as a decision-making model or because they are not formally introduced to other alternatives? Hardy indicates that role theory literature *per se* does not fully explore the range of strain-reducing strategies (including various bargaining techniques and symbolic interaction strategies).

Following is a representative log sample of a student developing a teacher role.

1/31–2/3   This week I contacted my first major conflict when viewing roles . . . a student had decided to work with a patient who after one month's hospitalization, was to have his leg amputated. Needless to say, he was very angry on his first postoperative day . . . he did such things as refuse medication, refuse to eat, refuse a bath, etc. . . . Within two hours the student was reduced to tears, and felt much of the patient's anger was due to her "being only a student." I spent time with her alone and then with her and the patient, which did encourage him to open up. Because of many pressures on the patient, I became more actively involved . . . I spent time role modeling behaviors with the patient, because I knew the student was unable to handle this kind of thing. In retrospect, I continue to find this experience very upsetting. I believe that in the teaching role it was my job to teach and my client was the student. Yet, I felt a strong obligation to the patient. . . . To analyze in terms of role theory, my role set was varied, going from staff, to preceptor, to student, to patient. All were sending me varied messages, most of them being evaluative, and those from especially the staff being negative. I also felt many pressures. Listed under the categorization suggested by Aradine and Denyes, *"Self-pressure"*: frustration with situation, philosophical conflict in what I feel the role of clinical instructor should be, interpersonal conflict with staff, *Systems Pressure*: quality of patient care given by others, system of team nursing . . ., *Role Pressure*: multiple stimuli, no peer to discuss this with at the time—no actual power, no authority in the situation. While all of this was going on, I left to develop my plan of action. I utilized a decision-making approach by listing the alternatives to the situation and decided to remain actively involved and consider my part as that of role model.

This process reflects the format followed by the majority of students in their logs: problem definition, search process, decision.

DOCTOR-NURSE CONFLICT

The third significant pattern reflected in the logs involves the relationships between medical and nursing staff. Smoyak writes:

The jurisdiction of nursing practice always has comprised the nurturing, caring, helping to cope, comforting, counseling, supporting activities in health care delivery. However, when nurses today do what only physicians did previously, conflict is generated.[5]

This is significant in examining doctor/nurse conflict, but another point made in the same article cautions that a nurse may be a victim of organizational illness and may cope by placing blame on the physician who, in return, responds in anger.

The following log documentation, selected as representative, reflects the socialization process for the further development of professional autonomy and increased accountability for the client. The student does attempt some analysis of organizational influence in her interactions. She also identifies aspects of jurisdiction of her practice.

2/7 . . . I got such an interesting reaction from the staff nurses at _____, when I told them what patient I have chosen to follow. I know they feel because I'm getting my master's degree I should be taking patients in ICU (only with complicated medical diagnosis). They have such a hard time with the fact that I don't choose these patients. It's kind of sad though that the nurses are not able to see the importance of nursing problems. Esteem and greatness (for them) is based on medical things.

2/13   I'm taking care of a child with fairly severe congenital heart disease whose medical condition at the time is stable, but who is not eating well for an unknown reason. She's not taking much with oral feedings and I know that soon the doctors will write an order for her to be tube fed—so—I did lots of research and came up with a new type of nipple that I feel should be tried. I presented my data to the resident on the case and told him I'd like to give the nipple a try. He responded "No, I don't like the idea." Me: "Why?" Him: "I just don't. Too much danger of aspiration. Tube feed her and stick with the regular nipple." Well I'm quite frustrated at this point. I know the resident has no good reason not to let me try the nipple. I know the harm that may be done with excessive tube feeding (which is what will happen with babies with feeding problems in large, busy institutions). It seems it can't hurt to try something new. Well at this point I was frustrated—I went to have coffee and thought about the situation. I decided the resident can't be expected to see feeding problems as a nursing problem because nurses in the insitution haven't got their stuff together and haven't identified it as such. And yet it is very definitely a nursing problem. Nurses feed the children 24 hours a day. Doctors come in, look and write orders. So—don't be angry with the doctor. Instead show him your commitment, concern and knowledge in this area. In the meantime (because it will be a long time before the resident's ideas will be changed) I'll go over his head and get permission from the staff MD, which is what I did, and he gave me full authority over the feeding program. It's gone well and the resident seems to be changing his attitude as time passes and I'm changing mine too.

3/8   I picked up a new patient today. I see Dr. _____ in the hall, he's the intern involved in the case. I recognize him because one of the staff had pointed him out to me earlier. I have an important piece of information to give him besides wanting to introduce myself. "Hi, Dr. A?" Dr.: "Yes" Me: "I'm a graduate student in nursing. I'm going to be working with you in taking care of _____." Dr: "Why?" (no eye contact, starts to walk away.) Me: "Dr. I wasn't through. I'm working with her because I think I can help the family and her with the feeding problem. I also wanted to tell you that the patient had a guaiac positive stool this morning, it smelled like blood also. . . ." Dr: "I guess we'll have to look into that." (leaves) Me: Go out to desk, chart is flagged for new orders—I look and see Dr. A. has written an order to d/c patient's IV. I wonder in view of the information I just gave him whether he'd like to change that order. I see him approaching the desk. "Oh, Dr. A., in view of the information I gave you, do you still want patient's IV d/c'd?" Dr: (looks irritated) "Yes, I wrote the order. We only have evidence of slow bleeding if any—even an IV won't help." Me: "O.K., I thought you might want to keep a line open for blood. If you're discontinuing the IV do you want her to be on oral ampicillin?" (has been receiving IV). Dr: "I don't know yet, Dear! We don't have the results from the sed cultures so I can't decide." (as he's talking he's crossing out the order to d/c the IV) Me: "Fine Dr., if you're busy I don't need to talk to you right now." (I'm really reacting emotionally with anger to the way I'm being talked to) Dr. walks away. Now I could have left it like this but I thought, "Dammit, I have to be able to work with this guy in order to help this patient," so I walked up to him in the hall. Me: "Hey Dr., I don't want to start out on the wrong foot with you. We have to be able to communicate with each other. I want you to know that I'll be asking lots of questions; it's my nature, it's the way I learn. I'm not questioning your orders." Dr: (face is red, can't seem to look in my eyes) "That's o.k., I don't mind questions." Me: "Good." So that's it and it should be straightened out, right? I have attempted to reconcile a bad start and to keep communication lines open. And yet, I feel uneasy about it. I also feel like, why does this seem to happen so often between doctors and nurses. What is the intern reacting to? Why do I seem to threaten him so much? (and I think I do). It seems like there shouldn't have to be so much extra in the way—before you get to patient care.

4/4 I'm surprised when I go back over what's been written here. So far much of it is about Dr./Nurse relationsips. I would never have admitted before this semester that I was bothered by this. It is good to get it down on paper and look at it.

4/30 Analyzing conflict situations in the detail used in the log is extremely helpful. I think it is a method I will continue to use. It allows for planning for round II; also I think by writing a situation down some of the emotion connected with the situation is dissipated. My attitudes regarding Dr./Nurse relationships have been tempered. I think just admitting I have some problems in this area has helped.

It should be noted that although conflict resolution has not taken place, the student has indicated she is now better able to examine her interactions rationally and has not been discouraged in her quest for change. As she notes, it has helped her prepare for future experiences.

SELF-REINTEGRATION

The fourth and last pattern reflected in student logs is the indication that by the end of the semester, students undergoing a socialization process in the advanced practitioner/teacher or practitioner/manager role are able to reintegrate themselves. The closure of logs reflect a more mature self within a new professional identity. The following excerpt is from the log of a student developing the practitioner role.

4/6   During the 3 months as my role ambiguity has decreased, I have been able to set some goals for myself concerning my future role development.   1.   I would like to continue to provide high quality nursing care to my caseload of clients as they move in and out of various health care settings.   2.   I would like to explore other ways of providing continuity of care to clients in the health care system to decrease the fragmentation of care that now exists.   3.   As I move from my limited scope of advanced practitioner, I am expanding my decision making from what Cleo Silver calls "programmed" to "unprogrammed." I feel the nurse practitioner is uniquely qualified to deal with complex health problems and their psychosocial ramifications.   4.   Role pressures are decreasing for a number of reasons: (a) the staff now has a role set for me and no longer feels threatened. (b) I have more specific expectations of them now that I have increased my understanding of the organization they function in. The mutual understanding of each other's role has opened up lines of communication and enabled me to accomplish things for my clients on the basis of my personal authority, although I do not have any formal authority with the organization.   5.   Role stress and strain have decreased as I have become socialized to the role of advanced practitioner and clarified my self expectations. Increasing my personal resources and using problem solving approaches (like working second shift part of the time) has lessened role strain considerably.   6.   Role conflict with the staff has decreased since I started attending their weekly staff meetings a month ago. Through communication we have discovered some common values and this has enabled us to establish a working relationship. The decrease in conflict has facilitated both my patient care and my change project on the unit.

Another closure statement in the log was made by a student with a teaching background concurrently taking an advanced practitioner practicum and the teaching practicum.

4/30   Log Closure Statement *Teacher Role.* This role is comfortable, but in analysis, probably the role in which lesser movement occurred from initial to terminal behaviors and expectations. Several factors influenced this statement, probably the most significant being a sense of prior socialization related to past experience. The frustrations met within this role were associated strongly with a discrepancy based on my expectations versus course content in general. This is the role I most probably will continue in a working environment to some degree. My immediate plans are to return to a teaching commitment at _____. However, I do recognize that this institutional structure by nature will present many "stresses" and will most likely not provide satisfaction for a long period of time. *Advanced Practitioner Role* Although this role is not as clear to me as the teacher role, I feel that the most personal growth has been within this area, especially in regard to the "subroles" of nurse as: advocate, collaborator, and humanizer. I'm also more strongly committed to the value of nursing research within advanced practice. In the beginning of the course, this role provided the sources of most stress which were resolved to a great extent. However, several limitations are recognized. For example, I didn't attempt to negotiate a role within a system, other than the "graduate student" role. If I had attempted such a role negotiation, I recognize that a whole other "stress arena" would have been engaged! One area of attitude change on my part is that I am now sure that I could not be long satisfied with any role that did not include some aspect of direct delivery of nursing care in a client situation . . . In general, I feel my overall response to stress has been in terms of a coping pattern directed primarily at the stressor, and through group support from faculty preceptors and fellow graduates. In terms of strategies for management of stress, the two target areas most heavily identified seem to be "focal person" as target and "role" as target with the "system" as target to a lesser degree [Kahn and Quinn].

In conclusion, over the two-year period of utilizing and refining the log as a teaching tool, several positive outcomes for students have been noted.

There has been an enhanced ability to focus on the process of role development, students are better able to clarify goals, and they approach their professional development process in a more analytical manner. Students have frequently reflected that they think the strategy of keeping a log is helpful enough to continue it during the initial phase of employment when implementing new nursing roles.

REFERENCES

1. Kahn, Robert and Quinn, Robert: *Role Stress: A Framework for Analysis.* In McLean, Alan (ed.): *Mental Health and Work Organizations.* Chicago, Rand McNally and Co., 1970; Aradine, Carolyn and Denyes, Mary Jean: Activities and pressures of clinical nurse specialists. *Nursing Research,* 21:411–418, September–October 1972; Kramer, Marlene and Schmalenberg, Claudia E.: Conflict: The cutting edge of growth. *Journal of Nursing Administration,* 6:19–25, October 1976; Filley, Alan: *Interpersonal Conflict Resolution.* Glenview, IL, Scott, Foresman and Co., 1975.
2. Kahn, Robert and Quinn, Robert: *Role Stress: A Framework for Analysis.* In McLean, Alan (ed.): *Mental Health and Work Organizations.* Chicago, Rand McNally and Co., 1970.
3. Aradine, Carolyne and Denyes, Mary Jean: Activities and pressures of clinical nurse specialists. *Nursing Research,* 21:411–418, September–October 1972.
4. Hardy, Margaret: Role stress and role strain. In Hardy, Margaret and Conway, Mary (eds.): *Role Theory Perspectives for Health Professionals.* New York, Appleton-Century-Crofts, 1978.
5. Smoyak, Shirley: Problems in interprofessional relations. In Chaska, Norma (ed.): *The Nursing Profession Views Through the Mist.* New York, McGraw-Hill Co., 1978, pp. 323–329.

BIBLIOGRAPHY

Aradine, Carolyn and Denyes, Mary Jean: Activities and pressures of clinical nurse specialists. *Nursing Research,* 21:411–418, September–October 1972.

Bailey, June and Claus, Karen: *Decision Making in Nursing Tools for Change.* St. Louis, C.V. Mosby Co., 1975.

Filley, Alan: *Interpersonal Conflict Resolution.* Glenview, IL, Scott, Foresman and Co., 1975.

Hardy, Margaret: Role stress and role strain. In Hardy, Margaret and Conway, Mary (eds.): *Role Theory Perspectives For Health Professionals.* New York, Appleton-Century-Crofts, 1978.

Kahn, Robert and Quinn, Robert: *Role Stress: A Framework for Analysis.* In McLean, Alan (ed.): *Mental Health and Work Organizations.* Chicago, Rand McNally and Co., 1970.

Kramer, Marlene and Schmalenberg, Claudia E.: Conflict: The cutting edge of growth. *Journal of Nursing Administration,* 6:19–25, October 1976.

Smoyak, Shirley: Problems in interprofessional relations. In Chaska, Norma (ed.): *The Nursing Profession Views Through the Mist.* New York, McGraw-Hill Co., 1978, pp. 323–329.

Suggested Reading

Socialization

Conway, Mary and Glass, Laurie: Socialization for survival in the academic world. *Nursing Outlook*, 26:424-429, 1978.

Gliebe, Werner: Faculty consensus as a socializing agent in professional education. *Nursing Research*, 26:428-431, November-December 1977.

Kramer, Marlene: Educational preparation for nurses roles. In *New Perspectives in Nursing Education*. St. Louis, C. V. Mosby, 1976, pp. 95-118.

Rosow, Irving: *Socialization Old Age*. Los Angeles, University of California Press, 1974. (Adult Socialization Theory)

Role Theory

Benner, Patricia and Kramer, Marlene: Role conceptions and integrative role behavior of nurses in special care and regular hospital units." *Nursing Research*, 21:20-29, January-February 1972.

Biddle, Bruce J. and Thomas, Edwin J.: *Role Theory: Concepts and Research*. New York, John Wiley and Sons, 1966.

Bryant, John H.: Health care trends and nursing roles. *Health Care Dimensions: Barriers and Facilitators to Quality Health Care*. Philadelphia, F.A. Davis, 17-28, 1975.

Cassidy, Jean E.: The advanced nursing practitioner: A dilemma for supervisors. *Journal of Nursing Administration*, 5:40-42, 1975.

Chaska, Norma: *The Nursing Profession Views Through the Mist*. New York, McGraw-Hill Co., 1978.

Christman, Luther: Educational Standards Versus Professional Performance. In *New Perspectives in Nursing Education*. St. Louis, C.V. Mosby, 1976, pp. 37-49, 1976.

Conway, Mary E.: Management effectiveness and the role making process. *Journal of Nursing Administration,* 4:25-28, 1974.

Grissum, Marlene and Spengler, Carol: *Womanpower and Health Care*. Boston, Little, Brown and Co., 1976.

Hardy, Margaret and Conway, Mary: *Role Theory Perspectives for Health Professionals*. New York, Appleton-Century-Crofts, 1978.

Keller, Nancy S: Private nursing practice: Some facilitators to quality health care. *Health Care Dimensions: Barriers and Facilitators to Quality Health Care*. Philadelphia, F.A. Davis Co., 1975.

Kramer, Marlene: Role models, role conception, and role deprivation. *Nursing Research*, 17:115-120, March-April 1968.

Kramer, Marlene: *Reality Shock. A Search for a Way Out*. St. Louis, C.V. Mosby, pp. 27-66, 1974.

Kramer, Marlene and Schmalenberg, Claudia: *Path to Biculturalism*. Wakefield, MA, Contemporary Publishing, Inc., 1977.

Kramer, Marlene, McDonnell, Catherine, and Reed, John L.: Self-actualization and role adaptation of baccalaureate degree nurses. *Nursing Research*, 21:111-123, March-April 1972.

Love, Lucille L.: The Process of Role Change. In Carlson, Carolyn (ed.): *Behavioral Concepts and Nursing Intervention*. Philadelphia, J.B. Lippincott, 1970.

Malaznik, Nancy: Theory of role function. In Roy, Sr. Callista (ed.): *Introduction to Nursing: An Adaptation Model*. Englewood Cliffs, Prentice-Hall, 1976.

Marwell, G. and Hagen, J.: The organization of role relationships: Systematic description. *American Sociological Review*, 35:884-900.

Meleis, Afaf Ibrahim: Role insufficiency and role supplementation: A conceptual framework. *Nursing Research*, 24:264-271, July-August, 1975.

Owens, Robert G.: Interpersonal Relations and Organizational Behavior. In *Organizational Behavior in Schools*. Englewood Cliffs, Prentice-Hall, 1970, pp. 66-68.

Padilla, G.V. *The Clinical Nurse Specialist: An Experiment in Role Effectiveness and Role Development*. Chap. IV. Duarte, Calif. City of Hope National Medical Center, pp. 32-49.

Riehl, J. and McVay, J.W: *The Clinical Nurse Specialist: Interpretation*. New York, Appleton-Century-Crofts, 1973.

U.S. Department of Health, Education and Welfare. *Role*. A Review and Evaluation of Nursing Productivity (Jelinck, Richard and Dennis, Lyman)

Systems

Claus, Karen and Bailey, June: *Power and Influence In Health Care*. St. Louis, C.V. Mosby Co., 1977.

Hoetker, James, Fichtenau, Robert and Farr, Helen L.K.: *Systems, Systems Approaches and the Teachers*. Urbana, IL, National Council of Teachers of English, 1962, pp. 1-22.

Leininger, Madeline: Health care delivery systems for tomorrow: Possibilities and guidelines. *Health Care Dimensions: Barriers and Facilitators to Quality Health Care*. Philadelphia, F.A. Davis, 1975.

Nadler, Gerald. *Work Systems Design: The Ideals Concept*. Homewood, IL, Irwin, Inc., 1967.

The Development of Identity

Becker, Howard S.: Personal change in adult life. In Benne, Warren G., Benne, Kenneth D., and Chin, Robert (eds.): *The Planning of Change*. 2nd ed. Chicago, Holt, Rinehart and Winston, Inc., 1969, pp. 255-267.

Erickson, Erik H.: *Identity Youth and Crisis*. New York, W.W. Norton, 1968.

Change/Change Agent

Asprec, Elsie Suajico: The process of change. *Supervisor Nurse*, 6:15-24, October 1975.

Bailey, June T. and Claus, Karen E.: *Decision Making in Nursing: Tools of Change*. St. Louis, C.V. Mosby, 1975.

Bennis, Warren G., Benne, Kenneth and Chin, Robert (eds.): *The Planning of Change*. 2nd ed. Chicago, Holt, Rinehart, and Winston, Inc., 1969.

Chin, Robert: The Utility of Systems Models and Developmental Models for Practitioners. In Bennis, Warren G., Benne, Kenneth D., and Chin, Robert (eds.): *The Planning of Change*. 2nd ed. Chicago, Holt, Rinehart and Winston, Inc. 1969, 297-312.

Epstein, Rhoda B.: Theory and process of change. *Coping with Change Through Assessment and Evaluation*. NLN Publication No. 23-1618. New York, NLN, 1976, pp. 1-12.

Havelock, Ronald G.: *The Change Agent's Guide to Innovation in Education*. New Jersey, Educational Technology Publications, 1973.

Kelman, Herbert C.: Manipulation of human behavior: An ethical dilemma for the social scientist. In Bennis, Warren C., Benne, Kenneth D., and Chin, Robert (eds.): *The Planning of Change*. 2nd ed., Chicago, Holt, Rinehart, and Winston, 1965, pp. 31-46.

Kreitlow, Burton: The Adult Educator as Change Agent. In Cooper, Signe (ed.): *Critical Issues in Continuing Education in Nursing*. Madison, University of Wisconsin, 1972, pp. 58-64.

Rogers, Janet A.: Theoretical considerations involved in the process of change. *Nursing Forum*, 12:2, 1973.

Silver, Cleo: The clinical specialist as a change agent. *Supervisor Nurse*, 4:19-27, September 1973.

Simeon, Shirley R.: Educators as change agents in the institution of nursing. *Journal of Continuing Education in Nursing*, 6:7-12, February 1975.

Stevens, Barbara J.: Effecting change. *Journal of Nursing Administration*, 5:23-26, February 1975.

Creative Problem Solving

Andrulis, Richard S.: A deeper look at creativity. *American Association of University Women Journal*, 40-43, April 1976.

Ashley, JoAnn and LaBelle, Beverly M.: Education for freeing minds. *New Perspectives in Nursing Education*. St. Louis, C.V. Mosby, 1976, pp. 50-75.

Frymier, Jack R.: Issues in perspective. *Theory Into Practice* 15:23-30, February 1976.

McDaniels, Michael A. and Mendell, Jay S.: What futurists can learn from creative problem solvers. *American Association of University Women Journal*, 38-40, November 1975.

Wong, Penelope, Doyle, Michael and Straus, David: Problem solving through process management. *Journal of Nursing Administration*, 5:37-39, January 1975.

Power/Autonomy

Ashley, Jo Ann: This I believe about power in nursing. *Nursing Outlook*, 21:10, October 1973.

Bowman, Rosemary Ameson and Culpepper, Rebecca Clark: Power: Rx for change. *American Journal of Nursing*, 74:1053-1056, 1974.

Maas, Meridean: Nurse Autonomy and Accountability in Organized Nursing Services. In Stone, Sandra, Berger, Marie Steng, Elhart, Dorothy, Firsich, Sharon Cannell and Jordan, Shelley Baney (eds.): *Management for Nurses: A Multidisciplinary Approach*. St. Louis, C.V. Mosby, pp. 34-48, 1976.

Zalesnik, Abraham: Power and Accountability: Power and Politics in Organizational Life. In Stone, S., (eds.): *Management for Nurses: A Multidisciplinary Approach*. St. Louis, C.V. Mosby, 1976, pp. 13-33.

Conflict/Conflict Resolution

Benne, Kenneth and Bennis, Warren: Role confusion and conflict in nursing, The role of the professional nurse. *American Journal of Nursing*, 59:196-198, February 1959.

Filley, Alan: *Interpersonal Conflict Resolution*. Glenview, IL., Scott, Foresman and Co., 1975.

Janis, Irving and Mann, Leon: Coping with decisional conflict. *American Scientist*, 64:657-667.

Kahn, Robert and Quinn, Robert: Role Stress. A Framework for Analysis. In McLean, Alan (ed.): *Mental Health and Work Organizations*. Chicago, Rand McNally and Co., 1970.

McDonnell, Catherine, Kramer, Marlene, and Leak, Allison: What would you do? *American Journal of Nursing*, 72:296-301, February 1972.

Schmalenberg, Claudia and Kramer, Marlene: Dreams and reality: Where do they meet? *Journal of Nursing Administration*, 6:35-43, June 1976.

Veninga, Robert: The management of conflict. *Journal of Nursing Administration*, 3:12-16, 1973.

Watson, Jean: The quasi-rational element in conflict. *Nursing Research*, 25:19-23, January-February 1976.

Williamson, J.A.: The conflict-producing role of the professionally socialized nurse-family member. *Nursing Forum*, 11:356, 1972.

11
Preparing the Practitioner as a Teacher of Nursing

A. Lorraine Wallenborn

The role of the teacher of nursing is a complex one in which many role components can be identified. For each role component, distinct role behaviors can be identified. The individual who fills the complex role of teacher and practitioner can suggest additional role components that must be added to her repertoire of behaviors. Each graduate student who wants to be a practitioner/teacher has a concept, from past experience, of the teacher's role, but graduate students of recent years have vague concepts of the practitioner/teacher's role because there have been no such role models in their past. Therefore, there are no clear-cut role expectations for the graduate student. This role of practitioner/teacher and the role expectations, then, must be learned. The nurse-educator is responsible for helping the student-teacher learn this new role with its many components as well as the behaviors appropriate for each component, and the expectations for the role components. This chapter describes how faculty members at one university used a role-oriented approach to develop a program of preparation for the teacher of nursing who would also be functioning as a practitioner.

To pursue a role-oriented approach to curriculum development, the faculty must take into account selected concepts about role. The role concepts presented here are derived primarily from Parsons and Shils[1] and from Sarbin.[2] Sarbin defines role as an organized set of behaviors that belong to an identifiable position. These behaviors, he says, are activated when the position is occupied.[3] In this study, the role to be discussed is that of the teacher in the practice discipline of nursing. The identified position is also that of teacher, but the actual position will be filled in a baccalaureate program of nursing after the student completes the graduate program.

A role is enacted in a social situation or structure. Parsons says that the most significant unit of social structure is not the person but the role.[4] In the social structure, the enactment of that role always occurs in the social context of complementary roles. A role is not enacted in isolation. The teacher role is enacted in the social context of teacher-learner and in the social structure of the classroom and clinical settings. One social setting for the students and teacher of nursing is usually the busy hospital ward in a highly complex social structure, where the teacher must interact with many individuals. Thus, in addition to the complementary roles of teacher and learner, there are many more such roles operating in this setting. These complementary roles may be filled by nursing students, their instructor, patients, their visitors, physicians, nurses, and other hospital employees. The student-teacher has the awesome responsibility of learning the many and varied role behaviors appropriate for enacting her role in this complex situation. She must also learn to be discriminative in identifying the role expectations held by the different individuals who fill the complementary roles and also the expectations required in different situations. Through the process of anticipatory socialization, the student-teacher learns expected roles or role components before holding a position. In this anticipatory socialization process, she has the benefit of a role model and coach, the teacher of nursing or her preceptor. It is generally recognized that learning by observing and by working closely with a model is both efficient and effective. The importance of the coach in role learning cannot be overemphasized, Sarbin says, for the coach detects mistakes, suggests a regimen of training, and in a variety of other ways aids the learner in mastering his role.[5]

How then did this faculty develop a program that was to become an integral portion of the masters degree curriculum to prepare nurses to assume the role of teacher? A portion of a graduate program is not developed in isolation. When the study of this portion was initiated, a curriculum study of both the undergraduate and graduate programs had been in progress. The philosophy of the college of nursing has been revised and the conceptual framework, applicable to both programs, was further developed. The concepts chosen served as the framework on which the overall graduate program was built. Selected concepts were used to guide the development of the teaching component of the graduate program. Objectives for the program were developed, which would reflect the concepts identified in the framework. In the study of the teaching component, overall program objectives relevant for teaching were identified, as follows:

The graduate is expected to demonstrate:

• Ability to utilize a conceptual framework as a guide for . . . teaching nursing consistent with a holistic view of man and a changing society.

- Ability to improve . . . teaching through the utilization of the research process.
- Ability to initiate, maintain, and promote intra- and interdisciplinary colleagueship . . . (in the teaching of nursing).
- Ability to design programs for . . . education.
- Competence for and socialization to the role of beginning teacher of nursing.
- Those personal characteristics appropriate for the beginning teacher of nursing.

A subcommittee of the faculty then discussed the question: "What are the roles the teacher of nursing is expected to fill?" or "What are the role components of the role of teacher of nursing?" In an earlier brainstorming session faculty had identified 47 potential role components graduates of the masters degree program could be expected to achieve. These components were then ranked in terms of importance. Those given a high ranking for the role of teacher, it is interesting to note, were communicator, helper, humanizer, educer, technician, demonstrator-presenter, counselor, resource agent, interpreter, and enabler. All of these components, except demonstrator-presenter, also received a high ranking for the role of practitioner. However, because they were not sufficiently specific for the role of a teacher, they were rejected when reviewed by the subcommittee. The seven role components then identified and selected were:

- Advanced practitioner
- Learning facilitator
- Faculty member of a baccalaureate program
- Curriculum builder
- Counselor/advisor
- Scholar/researcher
- Facilitator of group work

The seven role components selected by the subcommittee were then utilized to determine the competencies students need to develop to be able to function in the role of teacher. These competencies later served as bases for validating the terminal objectives for the teaching component.

With the conceptual framework, program objectives, teacher role components, and competencies serving as a foundation and giving direction, terminal objectives were developed for the teaching component. Progressive steps toward the student's achievement of these terminal objectives can be identified; therefore, level objectives for each objective were also developed. Minor changes were made in the terminal and level objectives after they were reviewed and evaluated by faculty and graduate students. The final version appears in Table 11.1.

At this stage McLane had completed her study.[6] McLane, a member of the faculty involved in the curriculum study of the graduate program, used a role-competency approach in her doctoral dissertation. She developed and refined competency statements for the roles of practitioner, teacher of nursing, and manager of nursing. These competencies, which were identified and validated in her study, were now available for use in this curriculum study. Each competency statement in the list of 63 was evaluated in terms of its relevancy for the preparation of teachers. The evaluation was based on the judgment of members of the subcommittee. Twenty-eight statements were found to meet this criterion of relevancy for the study of the teaching component. Selected examples of statements from McLane's study are as follows:

- Design (with learners) educational experiences that lead to achievement of desired objectives.
- Utilize basic tenets of major families of learning theory to create conditions in the environment that maximize learning.
- Utilize teaching strategies that involve the learner and his feelings in each learning situation.[7]

An attempt was then made to relate the 28 McLane competencies chosen to each of the eight objectives of the teaching component (shown in Table 11.1) and to the seven role components identified for the teaching role. Competencies related to the objectives and role components were identified, as were those that showed no relation. This provided a cross validation or method of evaluation for the objectives. In a related activity, a research assistant had carefully scrutinized the objectives of all graduate courses to identify McLane behaviors included in the existing curriculum. This information was available and selectively utilized by the committee, which was studying the teaching component.

The above activities led to a modification of the terminal objectives for the teaching component. These modified objectives were then presented to students who were asked to rate how well they believed they had achieved each of them. Their ratings were generally good. The objectives shown in Table 11.1 were then presented to and accepted by total faculty.

The primary purpose for developing objectives is to give direction for the selection of learning experiences for the students. The courses and the kinds of experiences provided for and available to students are briefly described.

In the teaching component, the student completes nine of the total of 36

Table 11.1   Terminal and Level Objectives for the Teaching Component in a Graduate Program in Nursing

A. Base strategies for instruction upon a conceptual framework for teaching/ learning.

Level One	Level Two
Explore the various theories of learning Define own value system Choose models consistent with own value system Explore various instructional strategies Explore research findings on instruction	Test selected aspects of own conceptual framework for teaching Utilize research findings in operationalizing conceptual framework Evaluate own ability to utilize selected instructional strategies

B. Set objectives for learning and design educational experiences that lead to achievement of these objectives.

Level One	Level Two
Develop objectives that give direction to successful achievement of learning Identify variety of educational experiences Identify appropriate tools or methods for evaluating achievement of objectives in differing learning situations Explore various patterns for organization of learning experiences Study innovative approaches to education and new instructional strategies	Select learning experiences designed to achieve a selected objective Assist student to formulate and achieve objectives for own learning in a clinical setting Evaluate effectiveness of learning experience chosen by self or by students Successful development of a unit of content

C. Assist students in the learning process:
  1. Set an environment conducive to learning:
      a. Analyze the environment in a learning situation
      b. Assess student's learning needs and readiness for learning
      c. Create conditions in the environment that maximize learning
      d. Establish helping relationships which foster disclosure of learner specific needs
      e. Evaluate own ability to stimulate a learning environment and to facilitate learning
  2. Assist student to establish objectives for learning, to select learning experiences, to evaluate achievement of objectives, and to assess growth:
      a. Utilize evaluation of assessed learning needs and readiness for learning to include students in goal-setting process

Table 11.1—Continued

---

   b. Assist student in the formulation of specific learning objectives
   c. Assist student to select and design learning experiences that lead to achievement of stated objectives
   d. Assist student to select teaching-learning strategies which have a high probability of success
   e. Assist students to evaluate the effectiveness of selected experiences in achieving specific outcomes
   f. Assist student to assess progress toward own objectives for learning

Level One	Level Two
Analyze components of an environment conducive to learning	Analyze the environment in a learning situation
Develop insight into the dynamics of teacher-student interaction	Evaluate own ability to stimulate a learning environment, to facilitate learning
Identify cues students give when ready or not ready to learn	Analyze own behavior in teacher-student interaction
Judge the worth and fitness of an objective	Test and evaluate effectiveness of innovative instructional strategies
Select learning experiences based on principles of learning	Evaluate ability to help student learn
Understand philosophy, principles, and methods of evaluation	Observe students for cues of readiness to learn
	Constructively criticize student's objectives
	Assist in the selection of learning experience in the clinical laboratory setting
	Participate with cooperating teacher in the evaluation of student's performance and progress

D. Serve as a role model for students in the practice of nursing

Level One	Level Two
Explore the influence of the behavior of an effective role model (the professional nurse in the practice setting) upon student learning	Observe and analyze the influence of a role model upon student behavior
	Evaluate the influence of own behavior in nurse-patient situation upon student learning

E. Evaluate own effectiveness and growth as a teacher

Level One	**Level Two**
Identify criteria for effectiveness in helping students learn Assess own personal characteristics and level of teaching ability Set objectives for own learning and growth	Seek assistance of cooperating teacher in periodic assessment of own level of teaching knowledge and ability Evaluate increasing effectiveness in helping students learn Determine the additional growth and learning needed

F. Participate in the study and improvement of the curriculum

Level One	**Level Two**
Demonstrate knowledge of the principles and process of curriculum development Demonstrate application of these principles to a preservice program of nursing Explore the nature of peer and hierarchical relationships in effecting curriculum change Understand the role of the faculty member in the curriculum development process	Participate with the cooperating teacher in ongoing curriculum development activities

G. Participate in the activities of the employing institution

Level One	**Level Two**
Explore the organizational and administrative framework of a university and the relationship of a nursing unit to the parent organization Identify the role of the faculty member in university activities and governance Discover the means by which university (and nursing) faculty can initiate and effect change Identify the role of the faculty member in the extended educational unit	Participate as appropriate with cooperating teacher in university activities

semester hours for the program. Four semester hours are allotted to the practicum or student teaching experience, and five to the two courses that normally precede the practicum. It is recomended but not required that the first course be the *Seminar in Curriculum*. In this course, the student, alone or in a group, goes through the process of developing a curriculum for a preservice baccalaureate program in nursing. In this process, the student explores the various learning and nursing theories, defines her own value system and beliefs, explores instructional strategies, develops objectives, identifies learning experiences, organizes the learning experiences in a pattern based on a conceptual framework, and determines methods for evaluating the curriculum. Seminar discussions include these and related topics, such as the faculty member's responsibility for participating in curriculum development activities.

The second course in the sequence is usually, but need not be, *Teaching in a Practice Discipline*. It is recommended that it precede the clinical teaching practicum, but it may be taken concurrently. Thus, there are no prerequisites. The topics for the weekly seminar discussion are selected jointly by teacher and students. Although the schedule is somewhat flexible, time is allotted to explore the major understandings needed by the teacher in a practice discipline. Each semester, the following topics, as well as others reflecting student interests, are included: the nature of learning, approaches to identifying and structuring content, instructional modes and media, principles of counseling and guidance, and the process of evaluation. Students read widely for each seminar discussion. In addition, using a personal conceptual framework for nursing as well as for teaching, each student is expected to develop a detailed instructional plan for a specified unit of study. That is, the student selects a unit of content, formulates objectives, identifies pertinent learning experiences (out of class, in class, and in the practice setting), suggests teaching strategies, and develops a blueprint for the evaluation of student achievement. Also, each student presents a "mini class" to her classmates or to the undergraduate students.

When these two courses are completed, the student will have achieved the level-one objectives (Table 11.1). Level two and terminal objectives for the teaching component of the masters degree program will be achieved when the *Teaching Practicum* is completed. This practicum, or student-teaching experience, is usually, but need not be, taken during the student's last semester. Also, it is usually preceded by the *Seminar in Curriculum* and by *Teaching in a Practice Discipline* but may be taken concurrently. This practicum is designed to assist the student to analyze and test her skills in guiding the learning of baccalaureate students. Each student teacher is assigned to work with a qualified faculty member (cooperating teacher) who is responsible for guiding baccalaureate students in a clinical practicum. Every effort is made to assign students to faculty members whose responsibilities are similar to the expressed interest areas of the student. The faculty member is responsible for providing, under her guidance, opportunities for the student-teacher to participate in representative activities of a teacher of nursing and college faculty member.

The teaching component does not stand alone in the program. The learning experiences of this component contribute to the achievement of overall program objectives, and other courses in the program contribute to the development of the teacher role. The teacher is expected by her students to be the role model for a professional nurse. The courses in the nursing major prepare the graduate for becoming the desired role model. The core course, *Role Development,* helps the student understand the process of role development. As this course is often taken concurrently with the teaching practicum, the student is able to apply the principles of role theory as she is learning the components of the teacher's role.

EVALUATION

Objectives not only give direction to the program but also serve to evaluate student performance as well as the program itself. To give further meaning to the objectives, critical indicators were developed for each objective. These indicators would describe the student's behavior at the completion of the sequence of courses in the teaching component if the student had satisfactorily achieved the objective. The committee used as resources the level objectives previously developed for each terminal objective and the McLane behaviors identified as relevant to determine the critical indicators for each objective. The critical indicators are shown in Table 11.2. When this task was completed an evaluation tool was developed. The tool is used by the students for their self-evaluation and by cooperating teachers to evaluate student performance when the teaching practicum, the terminal experience in the teaching component, is completed. The tool was actually designed for evaluating the effectiveness of the teaching component. The form to be completed by the student is presented in Table 11.2; the objectives tives and critical indicators are the basis for evaluation. The form to be completed by the cooperating teacher is similar to that of the student except for the instructions, which read:

Thoughtful opinions are essential to the evaluation process. A critical, constructive viewpoint can help a teacher grow in effectiveness. Because you have served as a cooperating teacher for a master student who has now completed all the courses designed to prepare her for a beginning position on a faculty, I am asking for your beliefs as to how well these courses have actually prepared her.

Table 11.2 Evaluation of Student-Teacher's Preparation

Evaluation Form

To be completed by the master student

Student opinions are essential to the evaluation process. A critical, constructive viewpoint can help teachers grow in effectiveness. Because you have now completed all of the courses designed to prepare you for a beginning position on a faculty, I am asking for your beliefs as to how well these courses have actually prepared you.

DIRECTIONS: The objectives for the teaching component of the graduate program are listed in the left-hand column (A-G). Critical indicators are included beneath each objective. You are asked to rate yourself on each *objective*, using the scale provided; the critical indicators should be used to help you determine how well the objective was met. In the space provided at the right of the paper, give an example of an incident or behavior that would help us determine why you rated yourself as you did.

OBJECTIVES	WP*	AP	PP	NO	Comments/Example
The graduate of the program is prepared to:					
A. Base strategies for instruction upon a conceptual framework for teaching/learning					
• Articulate own evolving conceptual framework for teaching/learning					
• Select teaching/learning strategies which are congruent with conceptual framework					
• Evaluate own ability to utilize instructional strategies based on conceptual framework					

B. Set objectives for learning and design educational experiences that lead to achievement of these objectives
- Develop objectives that give direction to successful achievement of learning
- Design (with learners) learning experiences that lead to achievement of these objectives
- Evaluate effectiveness of learning experience chosen by self or by students

C. Assist students in the learning process
1. Set an environment conducive to learning
   a. Analyze the environment in a learning situation
   b. Assess student's learning needs and readiness for learning
   c. Create conditions in the environment that maximize learning
   d. Establish helping relationships which foster disclosure of learner specific needs

Table 11.2—Continued

OBJECTIVES	WP*	AP	PP	NO	Comments/Example
e. Evaluate own ability to stimulate a learning environment and to facilitate learning					
2. Assist student to establish objectives for learning, to select learning experiences, to evaluate achievement of objectives, and to assess growth					
a. Utilize evaluation of assessed learning needs and readiness for learning to include students in goal-setting process					
b. Assist student in the formulation of specific learning objectives					
c. Assist student to select and design learning experiences that lead to achievement of stated objectives					
d. Assist student to select teaching-learning strategies which have a high probability of success					

   e. Assist students to evaluate
      the effectiveness of selected
      experiences in achieving
      specific outcomes
   f. Assist student to assess
      progress toward own objec-
      tives for learning
3. Evaluate student's growth
   a. Provide learners with infor-
      mation regarding progress
      toward (desired) goals
   b. Participate with cooperating
      teacher in the evaluation of
      student's performance and
      progress

D. Serve as role model for students in
   the practice of nursing
   • Observe and analyze the in-
     fluence of a role model (the pro-
     fessional nurse in the practice
     setting) upon student behavior
   • Evaluate the nurse-patient situa-
     tion upon student learning

E. Evaluate own effectiveness and
   growth as a teacher
   • Assess own personal
     characteristics and level of
     teaching ability

Table 11.2—Continued

OBJECTIVES	WP*	AP	PP	NO	Comments/Example
• Set objectives for own learning and growth					
• Seek peer evaluation of personal and professional competency					
• Utilize the findings of educational research to improve own teaching skills					
• Continuously seek clarification of congruency of own dominant value system and own teaching practices					
• Evaluate increasing effectiveness in helping students learn					
• Determine the additional growth and learning needed					
F. Participate in the study and improvement of the curriculum					
• Identify the role of the faculty member in the curriculum development process					
• Recognize the need to utilize change theory to effect curriculum revision					

- Evaluate issues and trends influencing the delivery of health care and the findings of educational research to suggest curriculum improvements

G. Participate in the activities of the employing institution
- Explore the relationship of the nursing unit to the university as the parent organization
- Identify the role of the faculty member in university activities and governance
- Identify the role of the faculty member in the extended educational unit

*WP-well prepared; AP-adequately prepared; PP-poorly prepared; NO-no opportunity to prepare

By June 1979, the tool had been administered five times. For the most part, the student-teacher's ratings correlated closely with those of her cooperating teacher. Most students feel they are well or adequately prepared to assume the behaviors described in the critical indicators. A weakness is noted, however, by a number of students in their achievement of the objective, "Participate in the activities of the employing institution."

In an effort to determine the relationship between the student's self-evaluation and the cooperating teacher's evaluation of the student's performance, an overall score was given to the ratings of the student enrolled in the teaching practicum in the Fall of 1977. A score was computed to show the difference between the student's self-rating and the cooperating teacher's rating of that student. The comparative responses, overall scores, and differences are shown in Table 11.3. In each case the differences are slight; teachers tended to rate a student's performance higher than the student did. Similar comparisons with similar results were made in the other four semesters the tool has been used.

In a student's program, it is difficult to provide the opportunity for complete freedom to experience the full responsibility of enacting the teacher role. Limited experiences are offered, but the master (cooperating) teacher maintains full responsibility. The student, therefore, finds it difficult, while still very much involved in the program, to evelute the effectiveness and usefulness of what she has learned. Evaluation of the program, then, is best made after the student has graduated, is employed as a teacher, and has had some time to become comfortable in her role as a teacher and faculty member. Such an evaluation was sought during this study from recent graduates. Those who had completed the experiences of the component and were employed in a teaching position were asked to complete a brief questionnaire. They were asked to explain their answers to the following two questions: (1) are there areas in which you believe your courses did not adequately prepare you for your *faculty and teaching* responsibilities and (2) do you have suggestions you believe would improve the teaching component of the curriculum?

There were six anonymous responses. As in the previous evaluation, the responses were positive, even though the questions were negatively worded. Although few graduates responded, their suggestions and comments are given, because other graduates may have similar needs if they were polled. Three respondents asked for the opportunity (or the requirement, for the opportunity is available if the student requests) to prepare and deliver a lecture to a group of 25 or more. Two asked for help in the "whole field of audiovisual aids": procurement and use of the various kinds of equipment, development of slides and transparencies, evaluation of available materials. Two suggested more content be included relative to the con-

Table 11.3 Teaching Component—Graduate Program Self and Cooperating Teacher Evaluation of Student-Teacher's Performance According to Objectives for Teaching Component, Fall 1977

Student Evaluation	A	B	C1	C2	C3	D	E	F	G	Overall Rating†	Difference††
Self evaluation	WP*	AP	WP	WP	AP	WP	WP	WP	WP	2.67	0.53
Teacher evaluation	AP	AP	AP		WP	WP	AP/NO	NO	AP	2.14	
Self evaluation	AP	WP	WP	WP	WP	WP	WP	WP	AP	2.76	-0.1
Teacher evaluation	WP	WP	WP	WP	WP	WP	A/WP	WP	AP/NO	3.86	
Self evaluation	WP	AP	AP	AP	AP	AP	A/WP	AP/NO	AP/NO	2.11	-0.04
Teacher evaluation	AP	A/WP	AP	WP	AP	AP	A/WP	AP/NO	AP/NO	2.15	
Self evaluation	WP	AP	WP	A/WP	WP	A/WP	WP	A/WP	AP/NO	2.54	-0.24
Teacher evaluation	WP	WP	WP	WP	WP	WP	WP	WP	AP	2.78	
Self evaluation	WP	A/WP	WP	A/WP	WP	WP	WP	A/PP	P/A/WP	2.63	-0.23
Teacher evaluation	WP	WP	WP	A/WP	WP	WP	A/WP/NO	NO	NO	2.86	
Self evaluation	WP	WP	WP	A/WP	WP	NO/AP	A/WP	P/WP	P/AP/WP	2.52	-0.3
Teacher evaluation	WP	A/WP	WP	A/WP	WP	WP	A/WP	NO	NO	2.82	
Self evaluation	AP	AP	AP	WP	WP	WP	WP	PP	WP	2.33	-0.55
Teacher evaluation	WP	WP	WP	WP	WP	WP	WP	AP	WP	2.88	
Self evaluation	WP	WP	WP	A/WP	A/WP	WP	A/WP	WP	WP	2.88	0.5
Teacher evaluation	A/WP	AP	WP	AP	A/WP	WP	AP	AP	A/WP	2.38	

*WP = well prepared; AP = adequately prepared; PP = poorly prepared; NO = No opportunity to observe.
†Numbers assigned as follows, WP = 3; AP = 2; PP = 1; NO = Not counted, from which a mean was derived.
††Student rating minus cooperating teacher rating.

cepts and practice of evaluation and measurement. One suggested that a valuable experience for the student-teacher would be to have full responsibility for the supervision and instruction of six to eight students for a short period of time, but under the guidance of the master teacher. Respondents wished to assure faculty that they were quite satisfied with their program. As one student noted:

> For the time we have, we already pack a great deal of needed experience and information into that.

The comments of another respondent are also quoted:

> The suggestions above in *no way* reflect dissatisfaction with the nursing program. The strongest suggestions and comments I could make would all emphasize my desire that the many excellent features of the program be retained. In particular, I think the courses in curriculum development, practice teaching, research, and theories of nursing are essential. . . . I have found that the theoretical and practical preparation for teaching received is far superior to that obtained by associates from other institutions.

Instructors are evaluated by students at the end of each course and use these evaluations to improve the course. Faculty members also receive impromptu and unsolicited evaluations from students, graduates, and their employers. These evaluations are not presented in this report for they were not utilized by the study committee.

In summary, evaluation of the teaching component, as noted in the assessments of a student-teacher's performance by herself and by her cooperating teachers and in the evaluation by graduates who are filling the role of teacher, has been overwhelmingly favorable. The results of this curriculum study suggest to faculty that the objectives for the teaching component are appropriate and realistic for preparing students to fill the role of teacher of nursing with confidence and competence and that the objectives are adequately met.

POST-MASTER'S CURRICULUM FOR TEACHERS OF NURSING

Although evaluations by students and graduates indicate that they have been well prepared to assume the role of teacher, faculty members believed that preparation for some of the teacher-role components could be improved by providing additional learning experiences. These additional learning experiences as well as those offered in the program described earlier in this chapter are also needed by masters graduates whose programs offered no educational courses. Machan (1978) further explained the need for additional preparation for teaching, as follows:

One of the major problems of graduate education for professional disciplines, particularly health disciplines, has been the need for higher degree graduates with multifaceted role preparation. While these disciplines must, by their nature, provide graduate education that focuses on and strengthens the professional practice, at the same time the disciplines are in great need of advanced practitioners with preparation for teaching . . . roles. The needs are so great that employers will fill teaching . . . positions with individuals having little or no preparation in these areas; or sometimes the individuals have some preparation as teachers . . . but are lacking the depth and insight that can only come from advanced preparation in the discipline itself.

To attempt to solve the problem by increasing the credit content of master's programs is not likely to succeed since students cannot afford the added burden of expense and time to prepare themselves adequately at pre-master's level. It is unfair to the student to create programs that are out of line with master's programs of other disciplines.[8]

Recognition of these needs for teacher preparation prompted the faculty to undertake a study to develop and propose a post-master's program of preparation for teaching in university programs of nursing. The program would lead to a specialist-in-education certificate, in keeping with current trends in education, as Putnam (1970) noted:

Numerous institutions have an established program of study for the degree or certificate of Education Specialist, often abbreviated as the Ed.S. Usually this is given for completion of 60 semester hours beyond the bachelor's degree. . . . The Ed.S., designed for specialists in education, is granted at a point between the master of education and the doctor of education degrees. The degree may be a terminal one or may be a base for doctoral study.[9]

A choice could have been made among other post-master's degrees offered in universities: the Ed.A., Advanced degree in Education; the AGC, Advanced Graduate Certificate; or CAGS, Certificate of Advanced Study, but this faculty chose the Ed.S., Specialist in Education. The program planned for this study sets, as an admission requirement, a master's degree in nursing. Thus, the certificate would be granted at a point between the master of science in nursing and the doctoral degree.

Discussions were held with persons in administrative positions in the School of Education to determine the potential feasibility of a post-master's preparation for teaching in a health discipline, to be offered jointly by the college of nursing and the school of education. Other health disciplines were expected to be interested in such a program, but they would become involved at a future date. The school of education administrators expressed an interest in the possible development of such a program.

With the above preliminary decisions made, the committee at the college of nursing undertook the curriculum study. The work completed in studies of the teaching component for the master's degree in nursing served as background material for this study. However, committee members recognized that the limited credits available in the master's program would not be a restricting factor in the post-master's program. Thus, they had the freedom to stage a brainstorming session to identify many potential roles or role components of nurse-teaching in a university setting. The following 13 components were finally selected:

Counselor/advisor
Scholar/researcher
Facilitator of group work
Role model
Change agent
Designer of systems
Intra- and interdisciplinary colleague
Humanizer
Learning facilitator
Member of a faculty
Curriculum builder
Evaluator of student growth
Educator

Later, it was noted that these role components fell logically into the following six areas for role focus: (1) faculty member, (2) learning facilitator, (3) evaluator, (4) curriculum builder, (5) researcher, and (6) practitioner. Using the 13 role components as guides, teaching component objectives, evaluations from student-teachers and graduates, and the advice and suggestions of qualified nurse educators, the committee developed objectives and critical indicators for the post-master's program for the preparation of teachers. It will be recalled that critical indicators describe the specific behaviors students will exhibit if objectives are achieved. These may also be called role behaviors. Content appropriate for the achievement of objectives was then identified. The relationship between this content, role components, and the objectives and critical indicators is shown in Table 11.4.

Courses offered in the School of Education, College of Nursing, and other University departments were then reviewed and evaluated to see if their content seemed appropriate for helping students achieve the objectives, critical indicators, and role components noted in Table 11.4. Learning experiences required to meet the objectives, which were not offered in current courses, were identified, and a tentative curriculum model then developed.

At this time, in order to explore the merit of continued study and development of the proposed curriculum, a meeting was held by administrative officials of the University, the College of Nursing, the School of Education, and the study committee members. As a result of this meeting, an *ad hoc* joint committee of faculty members from the School of Education and College of Nursing was formed. This committee was charged with the responsibility for producing a proposal for the post-master's program of teacher preparation. Once the proposal was accepted by both the faculty of the School of Education and that of the College of Nursing, it would then be presented to the Board of Graduate Studies for approval. The next step would be approval by the Academic Senate.

The *ad hoc* committee then studied and made revisions in the tentative curriculum model prepared by the nursing committee. The objectives, critical indicators, and revised model were then sent to each faculty member of the School of Education and the College of Nursing. Each was asked to evaluate the objectives and judge the feasibility of the program.

The suggestions were used to make minor revisions in the curriculum model, shown in Table 11.5. The model includes the six areas of role focus. Within each area reference is made to the objective(s) to be achieved by the experiences to be offered. The experiences are presented as courses currently offered at the university, and listing the title. Content for which no courses exist is also identified, and suggested credit allotment for each area is given. It is noted that for doctoral preparation, should the student wish to continue study beyond the certificate, additional credits would be required in the role focus of researcher. Of course, there would be other requirements for doctoral preparation which are not included in this model.

At this time, the program has not been implemented. This proposal, however, has merit for nursing and other practice disciplines, such as dentistry and medicine, for the preparation of teachers who can guide effectively the learning of future practitioners. The effective teacher is made, not born.

Table 11.4 Relationship Between Objectives, Role Components, and Content Selected for Post-Master's Preparation for Teaching

Objective and Critical Indicators	Role Component	Appropriate Content
Graduates of the program are prepared to:		
A. Demonstrate a general understanding of higher education as a discipline:	Member of a faculty Scholar/researcher Intra- and interdisciplinary colleague	Philosophies of education Philosophy of evaluation Adult Education Issues and trends in higher education
1. Develop a philosophy of higher education (teaching/learning)		
2. Evolve a philosophy for evaluation of learning by the adult		
3. Evaluate the significance of issues and trends in higher education for baccalaureate programs of nursing		
B. Base strategies for instruction on a philosophy of education and a conceptual framework for teaching/learning by:	Designer of systems Facilitator of group work Learning facilitator Role model	Theories of learning Adult education Teaching learning strategies Evaluation and self-evaluation
1. Developing and testing own conceptual framework for teaching/learning		

2. Utilizing teaching/learning strategies congruent with conceptual framework

3. Evaluating own ability to utilize instructional strategies based on conceptual framework

4. Evaluating the effect of these strategies on student learning

C. Set objectives for learning and design educational experiences that lead to achievement of these objectives:

1. Develop objectives that give direction to successful achievement of learning

2. Design (with learners) learning experiences that lead to achievement of these objectives

3. Evaluate the effectiveness of learning experiences chosen by self or by students

Learning facilitator
Counselor/advisor
Humanizer
Evaluator of student growth

Objective development
Helping students learn
Teaching/learning strategies
Evaluation
Audio-visual materials and their place in education

Table 11.4—Continued

Objective and Critical Indicator	Role Component	Appropriate Content
D. Assist students in the learning process: 1. Set an environment conducive to learning a. Analyze the environment in a learning situation b. Assess student's learning needs and readiness for learning c. Assist students to cope with stresses that inhibit their learning d. Create conditions in the environment that maximize learning e. Establish helping relationships which foster disclosure of learner specific needs	Facilitator of group work Role model Learning facilitator Humanizer	Group dynamics Characteristics of college students Principles of counseling and guidance Developmental task of adolescent and young adult Self evaluation Conditions of effective learning Theories of learning

f. Evaluate own ability to establish a learning environment to facilitate learning

2. Assist student to establish objectives for learning; to select learning experiences, to evaluate achievement of objectives, and to assess growth

a. Utilize evaluation of assessed learning needs and readiness for learning to include student in goal setting process

b. Assist student in the formulation of specific learning objectives

c. Assist student to select and design learning experiences that lead to achievement of stated objectives

d. Assist student to select teaching/learning strategies which have a high probability of success

Counselor/advisor
Learning facilitator
Humanizer
Evaluator of student growth
Designer of systems

Knowledge of discipline as nursing

Table 11.4—Continued

Objective and Critical Indicator	Role Component	Appropriate Content
e. Assist student to evaluate the effectiveness of selected experiences in achieving specific outcomes		
f. Assist students to assess progress toward own objectives for learning		
3. Evaluate student's growth	Evaluator	Philosophy of evaluation
a. Implement evaluation strategies that are congruent with own conceptual framework	Counselor/advisor	
b. Develop a plan for evaluation of achievement of course/experience objectives and of student growth		
c. Select evaluation/testing tools which are appropriate for the kind of learning being evaluated		

d. Develop and validate
   evaluation methods and
   tools

e. Interpret and utilize results
   of evaluation tools used

f. Provide learners with information regarding progress
   toward (desired) goals

E. Serve as a role model for students   Role model
   in the practice setting   Humanizer
                                        Knowledge of nursing

1. Observe and analyze the influence of a role model (the
   professional nurse in the practice setting) upon student
   behavior

2. Evaluate the influence of own
   behavior in nurse-patient situation upon student learning

Table 11.4—Continued

Objective and Critical Indicator	Role Component	Appropriate Content
F. Evaluate own effectiveness and growth as a teacher	Evaluator Scholar/researcher Educator	Self-evaluation
1. Assess own personal characteristics and level of teaching ability		
2. Set objectives for own learning and growth		
3. Seek peer evaluation of personal and professional competency		
4. Evaluate systematically congruency between own dominant value system and own teaching practice		
5. Utilize the findings of educational research to improve own teaching skills		
6. Collect and analyze data to evaluate effectiveness in helping students learn		

7. Determine the additional growth and learning needed

G. Participate in the study and improvement of instruction and the curriculum in nursing

1. Utilize analytical skills and research processes to contribute to body of knowledge of nursing education

2. Identify the role of the faculty member in the improvement of instruction and in the curriculum development process

3. Recognize the need to utilize change theory to effect curriculum improvement

4. Evaluate issues and trends influencing the delivery of health care and the findings of educational research to suggest instructional curriculum improvements

Curriculum builder
Member of a faculty
Change agent
Intra/interdisciplinary colleague
Scholar/researcher
Designer of systems
Educator
Facilitator of group work

Curriculum development and evaluation

Table 11.4—Continued

Objective and Critical Indicator	Role Component	Appropriate Content
H. Participate in the activities of the employing institution	Facilitator of group work Inter/intradisciplinary colleague Member of a faculty	Colleague Practices and procedures Academic freedom Tenure University governance
1. Investigate the governing policies and structure of a university		
2. Explore the relationship of the nursing unit to the university as the parent organization		
3. Identify the role of the faculty member in university activities and governance		
4. Identify the role of the faculty member in the extended educational unit		

Table 11.5   Post-Master's Preparation for Teaching—Curriculum Model

Total credits required = 24 selected from the following areas as indicated:

Area I Role Focus: Faculty Member	Area II Role Focus: Learning Facilitator	Area III Role Focus: Evaluator
Content for this area contributes to meeting objectives A and H.	Content for this area contributes to meeting objectives B, C, and D.	Content for this area contributes to meeting objective F.
Credits required = 3	*Credits required = 9*	*Credits required = 3*
Current problems in Amer. higher ed. Theories of administration Group dynamics Role development Content needed for which no courses exist: Issues on higher ed. Adult education Overview of philosophy of education Seminar on teaching (including content on academic freedom, tenure, professional ethics, teacher's role in university hierarchy, legal aspects)	A course in theories of learning* Theories of learning applied to instruction Effective college teaching Group dynamics Teaching in a practice discipline The contemporary college student Content needed for which no courses exist: Internship in college* Teaching (collaborating with college of nursing) Courses for college level education Counseling for teachers (existing courses do not speak to teacher's counseling role) Media Development and Use* 0 credit	Content needed for which no courses exist: Measurement of student progress Evaluation of self, others

Table 11.5—Continued

Area IV Role Focus: Curriculum Builder	Area V Role Focus: Researcher	Area VI Role Focus: Practitioner
Content for this area contributes to meeting objective G.	Content for this area contributes to meeting objectives F and G.	Content for this area contributes to meeting objective E.
Credits Required = 3 *Seminar in 　curriculum	*Credits required = 3* Nursing research* Design and methodology ?Nursing research 　colloquium * = 0 cr. 　(1 sem) Intermediate research 　and statistics Techniques and devices 　for quantification of 　evidence Correlation analysis 　of research data Statistical analysis 　and research design or Graduate level research 　courses from other 　departments (e.g., 　psych, soc.) ------------------------------ Doctoral requirement for 　this area: 9 credits Dissertation	Prerequisite to 　program: Proficiency at an 　advanced level 　of nursing practice

*Required course

REFERENCES

1. Parsons, Talcott and Shils, Edward A. (eds.): *Toward a General Theory of Action*. Cambridge, MA, Harvard University Press, 1951.
2. Sarbin, Theodore R. and Allen Vernon, L.: Role Theory. In Lindzey, G. and Aronson, E. (eds.): *The Handbook of Social Psychology*. 2nd ed. Reading, MA, Addison-Wesley Publishing Co., 1968, pp. 488–567.
3. Ibid., p. 545.
4. Parsons, p. 190.
5. Sarbin, p. 548.
6. McLane, Audrey M.: Core Competencies of Master's Prepared Nurses and Implications for Program Development, Ph.D. dissertation, Marquette University, 1975.
7. Ibid., p. 87.
8. Machan, Lorraine: Proposed Post-Master's Prepared Curriculum for Teachers of Nursing. H.E.W. Grant 5 D23 NU00038-03, Milwaukee, 1978.
9. Putnam, Howard: Suggested Intermediate Graduate Degree. In Lehrer, A. (ed.): *Leaders, Teacher and Learners in Academe: Partners in the Educational Process*. New York, Appleton-Century-Crofts, 1970, pp. 325.

Suggested Reading

Biddle, Bruce and Thomas, Edwin J. (eds.): *Role Theory: Concepts and Research*. New York, John Wiley & Sons, 1966.

Corrigan, Dean C. and Garland, Calden B.: Role Analysis Applied to Internship Processes. In *Internships in Teacher Education*, Forty-seventh Yearbook. Washington, D.C., Association for Student Teaching, 1968, pp. 91–104.

Cottrell, Leonard Jr.: The adjustment of the individual to his age and sex roles. *American Sociological Review*, 7:617–620, October 1942.

Fry, Maureen S.: An analysis of the role of a nurse educator. *Journal of Nursing Education*, 14:5–10, January 1975.

Getzels, J. W. and Guba, E. G.: The structure of roles and role conflict in the teaching situation. *Journal of Educational Sociology*, 29:30–40, September 1955.

Goode, William J.: A theory of role strain. *Ameriean Sociological Review*, 25:483–496, August 1960.

Machan, Lorraine: Proposed post-master's curriculum for teachers of nursing. H.E.W. Grant No. 5 D23 NU00038-03.

McLane, Audrey M.: Core competencies of master's prepared nurses and implications for program development. Ph.D. Dissertation, Marquette University, 1975.

Merton, Robert K.: The role-set: Problems in sociological theory. *The British Journal of Sociology*, 8:106–120, 1957.

O'Connor, Andrea B.: Sources of conflict for faculty members. *Journal of Nursing Education*, 17:35–38, May 1978.

Parsons, Talcott and Shils, Edward A. (eds.): *Toward A General Theory of Action*. Cambridge, Mass., Harvard University Press, 1951.

Pfnister, Allan O.: The Preparation of College Teachers. In Lehrer, S. (ed.): *Leaders, Teachers, and Learners in Academe: Partners in the Educational Process*. New York, Appleton-Century-Crofts, 1970, pp. 228–230.

Putnam, Howard.: Suggested intermediate graduate degree. In Lehrer, S. (ed.): *Leaders, Teachers and Learners in Acadame: Partners in the Educational Process*. New York, Appleton-Century-Crofts, 1970, pp. 325–326.

Reitman, Sandford W.: Role strain and the American teacher. *School Review,* 79:543-559, August 1971.

Rowse, Glenwood L., Howes, Nancy J. and Gustafson, David H.: Role based curriculum development in higher education. *Educational Technology,* 15:13-22, July 1975.

Sarbin, Theodore R. and Allen, Vernon L.: Role theory. In Lindzey, G. and Aronson, E. (eds.): *The Handbook of Social Psychology.* 2nd ed. Reading, Mass., Addison-Wesley Publishing Co., 1968, pp. 488-567.

Seaberg, Dorothy I.: *The Four Faces of Teaching: The Role of the Teacher in Humanizing Education.* Pacific Palisades, Cal., Goodyear Publishing Co., 1974.

Sorenson, A. Garth, Husek, T. R. and Yu, Constance: Divergent concepts of teacher role: An approach to the measurement of teacher effectiveness. *Journal of Educational Psychology,* 54:287-294, December 1963.

12
First Steps in the Making of a Practitioner/Teacher

Penny J. Goodyear

The development of the practitioner/teacher is a hearty assignment. People have high expectations of her upon the completion of her preparation. It follows that she must attend a good program that will foster the development of this role.

I believe that I was well prepared for such a role, and in the following pages I will evaluate the objectives for a teaching practicum of the program I attended. As I sought attainment of these nine objectives I was simultaneously attaining objectives for a practicum in the practitioner aspect of my role as practitioner/teacher. Prior to this I had completed a practicum involving patients with chronic illness. So in addition to learning about teaching I was also following a case load of patients with acute illness in the same setting in which I taught baccalaureate students.

Let me begin by examining my background. I was new to the practice of teaching. Other than teaching patients I had had no teaching experience. I had completed two courses of study on curriculum development and theory content of teaching in a practice discipline. With my new experience as teacher came the role pressure that can be identified when any new role is undertaken. I will identify those pressures in four categories: self, system, role and environment. Each of the four categories has more specific characteristics.

Self pressures
  -my inadequacy in dealing with students
  -my uncertainty of feelings about teaching
  -my unfamiliarity with cooperating teacher either as a person or professional

System pressures
-the staff on the unit did not know me and were justfiably curious and cautious
-the patient care systems, physical setting, schedules, staff relation-ships, attitudes toward students, student teachers, or the cooperating teacher were unfamiliar to me
-the working relationships shared between staff members were unknown to me

Role pressures
-confusion regarding the role of the graduate student
-uncertainty about the way in which others perceived my role
-uncertainty of the accepted ways to pursue developing my role
-anxiety from my desire to establish a good relationship with the staff, students and cooperating teacher that would help us all grow
-anxiety from my desire to demonstrate a genuine interest in each stu-dent

Interpersonal pressures
-the need to know students well enough to understand their personal goals
-the desire to establish my own legitimacy as a practitioner/teacher without threatening anyone
-my unfamiliarity with the key people on the unit and in the hospital

Many of these pressures can be alleviated by direct action. This was used as the strategy in most cases, such as in learning the physical set up of the nursing unit. A scavenger hunt was designed by the cooperating instructor. This served as an ice-breaker, helping me be more relaxed with the students while helping us all work off a little nervous tension and it was a pleasurable, creative way to accomplish the task of learning the unit rather than enduring a drab tour.

This strategy worked well with senior students but might not have been so effective with sophomores. For the senior student it allowed a certain degree of independence and self-direction. The sophomore baccalaureate student would have too many pressures on her at that point for it to be effective. The unstructured nature would have added anxiety instead of relieving it.

The curious element in dealing with these four categories of pressure was that it took less time to resolve the same types of pressure in other prac-ticums I had taken. I believe that this was due to the complexity of the prac-titioner/teacher role. In other practicums I was dealing with only the practi-tioner role.

The practitioner/teacher role is complex because it is very dynamic. The variables are multiplied greatly. In the combined role there are the expectations of the students, staff, faculty members, graduate student and patients. One must deal with virtually the entire staff and most of the patients. There is continuous contact, conflict and resolution.

As a student/practitioner, the focus remains on the development of yourself into a practitioner with varied responsibilities at various times. The additional roles of teacher, change agent and problem solver may come into play at one time, or become dormant until called upon. In the student/teacher/practitioner role it becomes even harder to delineate one role from another at a specific time. Not only do you add the dimension of the teacher role with its inherent role pressures, but you have the constant responsibility for facilitation of another person's role development at the same time.

With this introduction, let us turn to how the course objectives in a teacher practicum helped the practitioner/teacher role evolve in my experience.

OBJECTIVE 1. ASSESS THE LEARNING NEEDS OF INDIVIDUAL STUDENTS

There are several steps and/or degrees of mastering this objective. The first and most obvious is that you must know the student as a person in order to assess her learning needs. A role conflict comes into play here. The baccalaureate student sees you as a person her own age whom she would like to know. At the same time she keeps herself from getting too close. The students weren't sure whether I fit in as a student or as a teacher, assuming that there are two sides.

The strategy I used in dealing with this uncertainty lies in the realm of what Carl Rogers speaks of as a realness or genuineness necessary on the part of the teacher. Some of the specific actions I utilized were to elicit and help clarify the personal goals of each student in the group while sharing the goals I had made for my own learning. We discussed their expectations of me and mine of them. Through this discussion it was determined that my role included being a resource person, validating questions or actions students identified, working with my own case load as well as visiting the students' patients, observing students, observing the cooperating teacher, teaching and evaluating, to name a few.

The students with whom I had the opportunity to work were very mature and bright. They had previous experience with graduate students as part of their clinical group. However, they felt that my role was a more interesting part of nursing than they had previously experienced. There were six basic ways in which I assessed the learning needs of the students. They were:

-private conferences with each student
-direct observation of their performance
-attendance at the theory portion of the course
-evaluation of the clinical log kept by each student on a weekly basis
-through seminar discussion following each clinical week
-by continuous dialog with my cooperating teacher

OBJECTIVE 2. FORMULATE BEHAVIORAL OBJECTIVES WHICH REFLECT STUDENT NEEDS

This objective was accomplished on a weekly basis between the cooperating teacher and myself. It was done in a manner that reflected my needs as a student/practitioner/teacher. Each week I would determine how well my goals from the previous week had been met or could have been met more fully. My objectives were then either revised or repeated. New areas for exploration were continuously identified.

An important point here is that I did not spend time formulating behavioral objectives for each of the students. They determined their own objectives. I found the students to be more critical of their capabilities than I would have been. This was more meaningful to them because they were directing their own learning. We were facilitating that process while fostering self-direction and critical thinking.

OBJECTIVE 3. SELECT LEARNING EXPERIENCES TO MEET STATED OBJECTIVES

This was probably the easiest objective to achieve. The clinical unit was extremely rich with opportunities for the undergraduate students to use skills and concepts and develop good staff-student relationships. It was much easier for them to concentrate on their objectives when the attitude of the staff was non-threatening. This, of course, was due to years of careful preparation and adjustment by my cooperating instructor. Things were not always calm, but were far more complacent than I had expected or been a party to in my experience as a staff nurse.

Assignment of patients was done the day before the students were expected on the unit. This was either done by the cooperating instructor, by myself, or together. The students were given assignments in several different ways. Many times the students had one, two, or three patients depending on their goals. Occasionally two students would be assigned to one patient if the needs of the patient were multiple or complex. Each of the patients was visited, if possible, prior to being assigned to a student.

The students benefit from this by getting a varied and challenging assignment and the staff benefits by having a lighter load, leaving some free time for staff development, inservice or conferences. The graduate student benefits by having multiple possibilities for observations of students in various situations.

The students were free to change their assignments if they felt it did not meet their needs, was too heavy or light, or if they had a particular patient in mind. They had to contact the instructor, explain, and clear it with the nurse-in-charge so the communication was clear to the staff, student, and patient(s) prior to the clinical laboratory period.

OBJECTIVE 4. GUIDE STUDENTS IN ACQUISITION OF NEW UNDERSTANDINGS, CONCEPTS, AND SKILLS

Clinical conferences were held at least weekly. During this time each undergraduate student presented a topic of her choosing which showed relevance to a new area of interest in nursing. Such things as nursing diagnoses, nursing theory, specific disorders and/or treatments were discussed. I gave two conferences. Their participation in the group process as well as presentation was considered. This was a time when we could collaborate, share, and explore.

On the clinical unit in their direct patient care and student-staff relationships there were also many instances to guide students to new concepts, understandings, and skills.

Time is a very real role pressure in the practitioner/teacher role. Often there was a strong urge to use a method or procedure with which I was comfortable instead of letting the student work it out for herself. This is a role conflict. The important thing, and possibly one of the most difficult to attain, is that the teacher aspect of the practitioner/teacher role must win out. More clearly, the priority in each case must be the student and his or her learning for the maximum benefit of the patient. It is a case of using a planned intervention rather than an instinctive strategy.

OBJECTIVE 5. USE OF A VARIETY OF INSTRUCTIONAL STRATEGIES

The biggest achievement that I see in the attainment of this objective was in exposing myself and the students to the practitioner/teacher role. Several of the students were thrilled with the fact that I also cared for and was responsible to patients. The students asked a lot of questions about my patients and many small patient care conferences were stimulated by their inquisitiveness. Many times the outcome improved strategies for our patient care in some small way.

The exposure to the demonstration of the practitioner/teacher role also helped to bridge the gap between expoundings of nursing educators and what nursing service demonstrated. I was an evolving role model. I began with great uncertainty just as each of the students did. I grew in my courage to use my skills and ideas just as they did.

OBJECTIVE 6. EVALUATE STUDENT PROGRESS

The evaluation of students was an on-going process. It was a cooperative effort on the part of myself, the student, faculty, and the cooperating teacher. In this area the students benefited to a great degree. Through their own contributions in the evaluation process the students were able to grow at their own pace. They were their own worst critics and more often than not, the staff, the cooperating teacher, and I needed to help the student be more realistic with her expectations about herself. It was amazing how many times a small positive accomplishment was an effective tool.

One area that could have used more attention is that of evaluation of communication skills. The students are usually quite capable of communicating with their patients. They do have difficulty in communicating with nursing and medical staff both in writing and verbally. This is probably one area that causes reality shock after graduation.

I do not feel I had adequate time or guidance to explore this. Even in the one extensive project that each of the students did there were many grammatical errors. True, these are non-nursing areas, but the end result certainly affects nursing. If we cannot put ourselves across as articulate professionals we will not be regarded highly. I believe this is important chiefly because of the esteemed position held by physicians. If we are to share a true collegial relationship we must present ourselves in a good light. We have a tough act to follow. Nursing must *earn* a place next to the other professional staff.

OBJECTIVE 7. ATTEND DEPARTMENTAL MEETINGS (AT LEAST ONE)

This was only required once during the semester. Frankly, I found it useless. We should either attend several or none. This again is limited because of time available. There are many conflicts that need to be worked out in a faculty department. This is a very real pressure to which any new practitioner/teacher will be exposed. Because the students' needs are of primary importance, these real aspects take "a back seat."

OBJECTIVE 8. ATTEND FORMAL CLASSES

After completion of my clinical teaching practicum I realized that there are time limits that are the most restrictive. Not only do I wish I had been able to afford more time to attend formal classes, but I also wish we had been able to try teaching a portion of one. We were required to do a video-tape on a subject of our choice. I believe that facing the critical eyes of undergraduate students would be better experience than facing a video-tape camera. It would also lessen the reality shock when a beginning teacher does some formal classroom teaching.

OBJECTIVE 9. OBSERVE THE COOPERATING TEACHER IN HER ROLE AS FACULTY MEMBER

The last objective was easily accomplished through many instances. The only way I could see an improvement in this area would be if it were to observe a practitioner/teacher at work.

In the beginning there were attempts to discourage me from taking two clinical practicums at the same time. The demands from these two courses were heavy. It was also an extremely realistic example of the work load most practitioner/teachers take on. I am glad I did take the challenge in this manner.

I could identify three areas of change in the nursing staff on the floor. The first change was in attitude. In my experience in other courses, the staff usually remained non-commital at best. Previously, after repeated attempts on my part to legitimize my presence, the environment remained strictly tolerant. In this instance, as a practitioner/teacher, the initial pattern was no different. The difference is that it grew beyond this. Instead of the tolerance there was no collegial relationship. The staff did not see me there briefly or sporadically to offer a lot of psychosocial suggestions. I was demonstrating an ability to care for patients and guide students in my unique way and make it quite clear I was open to their critique. The difference may have been due to my own strategies and approaches but I feel it was the combined role that gave the staff a different view of me.

I took some of the more difficult patients into my case loads and made sure the staff had as much feedback as I could supply. In one case it included following a very ill patient to another hospital and insuring the continuity of his case. The nursing staff saw this as a unique way to keep in contact with this man. I became a member of their team. This also carried over to their relationship with the students. I became a liaison. I was "one of them" and "one of us."

The second change was in interest. Instead of merely tolerating my presence, there were inquiries about my patients, offered bits of information, helpful hints and occasionally a criticism which was most timely but helpful.

The third change was in respect. The team leaders treated me as a true colleague and were quite open. They even had inquiries about my opinion on things. Two of them were anxious to see if I thought they could "make it" through the graduate program. This change was very welcome in that it provided me with a great deal of professional support. I also saw their inquiries as a vote of confidence in my abilities.

In summary I would like to say that I think the program described in this chapter is a sound one. It is not faultless or foolproof. It does provide the opportunity for growth. My specific interest was in getting a taste of the practitioner/teacher role before I needed to implement it.

13

Challenges for Continuing Education

Lorraine Machan and Madeline Musante Wake

The need for an integrated practitioner/teacher role presents challenges to continuing education. One of these challenges is to provide for the practitioner-teacher's continued professional development. Another is assuring that the faculty for continuing education, both in staff development and university settings, are truly competent in nursing practice and in teaching.

Because the concept of continuing education encompasses all levels of nursing practice, it is a powerful medium for changes in the profession. It can become an effective pathway to the production of high-quality practitioner/teachers. However, at this time, we know of no continuing education program that designs courses with this multifaceted role specifically in mind. A role-oriented continuing education curriculum could facilitate further professional growth for academically prepared practitioner/teachers and also enhance the practitioner's role effectiveness by adding teaching competence and the teacher's role effectiveness by adding practice competence, and both roles would be enhanced by research competence. The four chapters preceding this one can offer guidelines for developing such a curriculum.

Our continuing education department has instituted several steps in this direction by offering courses geared to master's level nurses. In one such course, Advanced Diabetes Care, the teachers were experts in areas of exercise, nutrition, and nursing care of the child and the adult with diabetes. Each of the four teachers in this series discussed recent research findings and their implications for practice. While this approach is important in so far as it facilitates the translation of research results to improved practice, it could be carried further by assisting practitioners in the design of meaningful data collection tools to test in practice settings the validity of published research, particularly since there is a growing body of evidence to support the concept of biochemical individuality. It could also facilitate the growth of the practitioner in diabetes care by offering courses of guided practice in clinical settings such as the ambulatory clinic described by Judith Miller in Chapter 4. In addition, it could provide instruction in the development of teaching materials for students at various levels, as well as for patients and their families.

Another approach used in our continuing education department is Clinical Nursing Symposia, a two-day program format (various program topics) that brings together expert practitioners with common interests. At a recent symposium on Neurological Nursing experts from two universities and two medical centers had been invited to discuss and integrate knowledge in this area of practice. This practice format not only develops the knowledge base of course participants, but also brings together practitioner/teachers in a given field who can mutually benefit from each other's expertise. This approach, therefore, is one method of continuing education instruction for the functioning practitioner/teacher. By sharing in discussions with other experts in the same field as continuing education faculty, the practitioner/teacher finds that teaching courses in continuing education is an experience in self-growth and learning. Continuing education offers a unique opportunity to test out concepts with groups of practicing nurses. It also opens the door for collaborative research projects by bringing experts together.

THE CLINICAL NURSE-SPECIALIST AS TEACHER

Clinical nurse-specialists demonstrate their expertise in a variety of settings and positions. At times, a lack of teaching skills can restrict the scope of a clinical specialist's impact on nursing practice in an agency or community. Our department is committed to facilitate the sharing of knowledge among clinical nurse-specialists. If the practitioner is to be a practitioner/teacher, she must be given the opportunity to develop the teaching aspect of her role. Rush University helps its faculty to develop and to improve their teaching techniques by providing a team of educational experts to assist them whenever they need and want help.

In our continuing education department, we recruit specialists whose expertise corresponds to the learning needs of our client group and help them to acquire and develop teaching skills. A specialist who has no experience as a teacher is coached by an experienced continuing educator. This coaching includes the collaborative design of learning experiences; guided experience in the use of various teaching methods, such as lectures, small group discussions, and panels; and a critique and evaluation by experienced teachers and participants.

STAFF DEVELOPMENT

Ideally, the staff development instructor should be a practitioner/teacher. However, too often one or both aspects of the role are deficient. Often a staff nurse who achieves well is promoted out of the nursing practice which is her strength. As an instructor, therefore, she loses her expertise and its currency, thereby contributing to the practice-education gap within a service setting. Also, the excellent clinician does not become a teacher simply by changing her title to "instructor." She needs a planned program for development.

The trend toward clinically based instructors for inservice education supports the practitioner/teacher philosophy. One Milwaukee hospital uses a centralized inservice staff as instructors in their routine orientation and procedural programs and a decentralized unit-based contingent for clinical staff development. The unit-based instructor is a nurse with demonstrated clinical expertise who has developed teaching competence. This nurse spends a certain percentage of her time in direct patient care so that the course content and skills she teaches are current and realistic.

RESEARCH PROMOTION

Research can be promoted and taught in specific continuing education courses or by including research methods and techniques in other courses. For example, we have offered courses that teach techniques in an experimental design format, e.g., tension-control techniques in which participants monitor each other's vital signs before and after each technique is practiced. Even though the data the group collects are not valid, the exercise provides an opportunity to explain how controls can be established and gives the nurses insight into themselves. The course encourages participants to collect data over a period of time, and to stimulate their interest, each participant is sent a copy of the tabulated data from all participants, along with a follow-up questionnaire designed to assess how they are using the knowledge they gained in the course.

As an example of how research can be promoted, the coordinator of a course on the Nutritional Needs of the Hospitalized Patient asked participants of the course to study the level of nutritional needs of clients in their agencies by collecting data to share with other participants. Groups of course participants would then discuss these client needs and develop a plan to improve the nutritional status of patients in their hospitals. Although this method lacks sophistication, it does illustrate the potential for nursing practice research in continuing education.

As functioning master's-prepared practitioners are increasing in numbers, efforts must be made, through continuing education, to build on the research skills and interests developed in graduate school. Some of these graduates are quite competent to design and teach introductory research courses for staff nurses and to carry out, with these nurses, small research projects relevant to improving their nursing practice. Even though there may be a trend toward clinically based instructors in staff development, research skills on the whole have not been given much attention. "Continuing education simply must take on some of the responsibility for preparing people to do studies, especially since such small percentages of nurses go on for higher education that prepares them for research."[1] The reader is also referred to Stevenson's chapter on Developing Research Potential in Part II of this book.

Wherever there are teachers of nursing, the relationship between practice, research, and teaching should be apparent. Wherever there are teachers of nursing, if the spirit and philosophy of "practice what you teach" prevails, the gap between service and education will disappear.

REFERENCE

1. Diers, Donna: The role of continuing education in promoting research in practice. *The Journal of Continuing Education in Nursing,* 8:54–62, May-June, 1977.

Index